Official Organ of the European Society for Paediatric Endocrinology

Hormone Research

International Journal of Experimental and Clinical Endocrinology

Founded 1970 as 'Hormones' by M. Marois

KARGER

Printed in Switzerland
on acid-free paper by
Thür AG Offsetdruck, Pratteln

Appears monthly:
2 volumes per year (12 issues)

Hormone Research

'Hormone Research' aims to provide rapid publication of clinical investigations and case reports, as well as experimental and methodological work related to endocrinology. Correspondence is welcome, but publication of letters is at the discretion of the editors.

Submission: Only original papers written in English are considered and should be sent to:

S. Karger AG
Editorial Dept. 'Hormone Research'
P.O. Box
CH–4009 Basel (Switzerland)

Manuscripts should be submitted in triplicate (with three sets of illustrations of which one is an original), typewritten double-spaced on one side of the paper, with a wide margin.

Conditions: All manuscripts are subject to editorial review. Manuscripts are received with the explicit understanding that they are not under simultaneous consideration by any other publication. Submission of an article for publication implies the transfer of the copyright from the author to the publisher upon acceptance. Accepted papers become the permanent property of 'Hormone Research' and may not be reproduced by any means, in whole or in part, without the written consent of the publisher. It is the author's responsibility to obtain permission to reproduce illustrations, tables, etc. from other publications.

Arrangement:
Title page: The first page of each paper should indicate the title (main title underlined), the authors' names, and the institute where the work was conducted. A short title for use as running head as well as the full address of the author to whom correspondence should be sent are also required.
Full address: The exact postal address complete with postal code must be given at the bottom of the title page. Please also supply Phone and Fax numbers.
Key words: For indexing purposes, a list of 3–10 key words in English is essential.
Abstract: Each paper needs an abstract of up to 10 lines.
Small type: Paragraphs which can or must be set in smaller type (case histories, test methods, etc.) should be indicated with a 'p' (petit) in the margin on the left-hand side.
Footnotes: Avoid footnotes. When essential, they are numbered consecutively and typed at the foot of the appropriate page.
Tables and illustrations: Tables and illustrations (both numbered in Arabic numerals) should be prepared on separate sheets. Tables require a heading and figures a legend, also prepared on a separate sheet. For the reproduction of illustrations, only good drawings and original photographs can be accepted; negatives or photocopies cannot be used. When possible, group several illustrations on one block for reproduction (max. size 181 × 223 mm) or provide crop marks. On the back of each illustration, indicate its number, the author's name, and 'top'. Color illustrations are reproduced at the author's expense.
References: In the text identify references by Arabic numerals [in square brackets]. Material submitted for publication but not yet accepted should be noted as 'unpublished data' and not be included in the reference list. The list of references should include only those publications which are cited in the text. Do not alphabetize; number references in the order in which they are first mentioned in the text. The surnames of the authors followed by initials should be given. There should be no punctuation other than a comma to separate the authors. Cite all authors, 'et al' is not sufficient. Abbreviate journal names according to the Index Medicus system. (Also see International Committee of Medical Journal Editors: Uniform requirements for manuscripts submitted to biomedical journals. Br Med J 1988;296: 401–405.)
Examples
(a) Papers published in periodicals: Kauffman HF, van der Heide S, Beaumont F, Blok H, de Vries K: Class-specific antibody determination against *Aspergillus fumigatus* by means of the enzyme-linked immunosorbent assay. III. Comparative study: IgG, IgA, IgM ELISA titers, precipitating antibodies and IgE binding after fractionation of the antigen. Int Arch Allergy Appl Immunol 1986;80:300–306.
(b) Monographs: Matthews DE, Farewell VT: Using and Understanding Medical Statistics. Basel, Karger, 1985.
(c) Edited books: Hardy WD Jr, Essex M: FeLV-induced feline acquired immune deficiency syndrome: A model for human AIDS;in Klein E (ed): Acquired Immunodeficiency Syndrome. Prog Allergy. Basel, Karger, 1986, vol 37, pp 353–376.
Further details: Authors may consult our leaflet 'Rules for the Preparation of Manuscripts', available on request from the Publisher, S. Karger AG, P.O. Box, CH–4009 Basel (Switzerland).

Page charges: There is no page charge for papers of 4 or fewer printed pages (including tables, illustrations and references). Each additional complete or partial page is charged to the author at SFr. 415.–/ US$ 275.00. The allotted size of a paper is equal to approx. 12 manuscript pages (including tables, illustrations and references). As the page charges are waived in any case for the first paper each year to be published by a member of ESPE, authors who are members of the ESPE should so indicate on the title page.

Galley proofs: Unless indicated otherwise, galley proofs are sent to the first-named author and should be returned with the least possible delay. Alterations made in galley proofs, other than the correction of printer's errors, are charged to the author. No page proofs are supplied.

Reprints: Order forms and a price list are sent with the galley proofs. Orders submitted after the issue is printed are subject to considerably higher prices. Allow five weeks from date of publication for delivery of reprints.

KARGER

General Information

Hormone Research

Publication data: 'Hormone Research' is published 12 times annually. Volumes 37–38 with 6 issues each appear in 1992

Subscription rates: Subscriptions run for a full calendar year Prices are given per volume, surface postage included.

Personal subscription: SFr. 278.60, US$ 186.20.
(Must be in the name of, billed to, and paid by an individual. Order must be marked 'personal subscription'.)

Institutional subscription:
(Regular rate.) SFr. 398.–, US$ 266.00.

Members of the European Society of Paediatric
Endocrinology: SFr. 76.40, US$ 51.05.
Lawson Wilkins Society; ISGD;
Schweizerische Gesellschaft für
Endokrinologie: SFr. 238.80, US$ 159.60.

Airmail postage: SFr. 35.–, US$ 30.00.
(Extra per volume.)

Microform subscription: SFr. 199.–, US$ 133.00.
(Available exclusively to subscribers of the paper edition.)

Single issues and back volumes: Information on availability and prices can be obtained through the Publisher.

Advertising: Correspondence and rate requests should be addressed to the Publisher.

Subscription orders: Orders can be placed at agencies, bookstores, directly with the Publisher S. Karger AG, P.O. Box, CH–4009 Basel (Switzerland)
or with any of the following distributors:

Deutschland:
S. Karger GmbH, Lörracher Strasse 16A
Postfach, D-W–7800 Freiburg

France: Librairie Luginbühl
36, bd de Latour-Maubourg, F–75007 Paris

Great Britain, Ireland:
S. Karger Publishers, 11 Ravenscroft Road
Beckenham, Kent BR3 4TP

USA: S. Karger Publishers, Inc.
26 West Avon Road, P.O. Box 529
Farmington, CT 06085

India, Bangladesh, Sri Lanka:
S. Karger India Subscription Agency
B–5/132 Safdarjung Enclave
New Delhi-110029

Japan: Katakura Libri, Inc.
36-9 Hongo 3-chome, Bunkyo-ku, Tokyo 113

Change of address: Both old and new address should be stated and sent to the subscription source.

Bibliographic indices: This journal is regularly listed in bibliographic services, including *Current Contents®*.

Book Reviews: Books are accepted for review by special agreement.

Guidelines for Disk Submission

Karger Publishers welcomes the submission of manuscripts on disk.

Please observe the 'Instructions to authors' as well as the following guidelines:

Technical Data

The preferred **storage medium** is a 3.5- or 5.25-inch disk in MS-DOS format. Macintosh is also acceptable.

The preferred **word processing package** is Microsoft Word. Other commonly used PC text programs are also accepted, as well as ASCII formats.

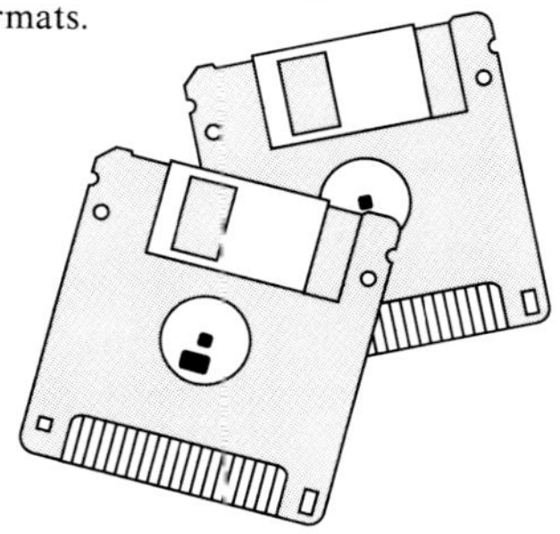

Handling

All manuscripts accepted for Karger publications are subject to copy editing. It is therefore essential that you send us a **double-spaced printout** of your manuscript which exactly matches the disk.

Any subsequent revised versions should be clearly marked as such, both on the disk and on the manuscript.

The copy-edited manuscript and the disk will be returned to you along with the galley proofs. Please be sure to **check the galleys against the manuscript** in which changes introduced by the copy editor and/or questions will be marked.

Please **label** your disk with (a) the title of the journal for which it is submitted, (b) a short version of the paper title, (c) your name and (d) the software and hardware used.

Text Arrangement

Text and headings should be ranged left throughout, without word breaks. **Do not center, space, or use block letters** for text and headings (except for abbreviations).

Do not use indentations to mark the beginning of a paragraph, but use one blank line between paragraphs.

Be sure to use the **same type style for headings of the same ranking** throughout the text.

When using **special characters** not available on a standard keyboard (including Greek characters), please do so by a readily identifiable code, and use the same code throughout the manuscript. Supply a **complete list of the codes used** at the beginning of the text.

Illustrations, tables and mathematical formulae will be handled conventionally.

KARGER

VIII International Symposium on Endocrinology and Development

Multiple Endocrine Diseases:
Growth Hormone Action:
Intersexuality

Telfs, Austria
October 11–12, 1991

Guest Editor
A. Attanasio, Bad Homburg

41 figures, 14 tables, 1992

KARGER

Hormone Research
Vol. 38, Supplement 2, 1992

Meeting and publication sponsored by
Eli Lilly International Corporation

S. Karger
Medical and Scientific Publishers
Basel · Freiburg · Paris · London
New York · New Delhi · Bangkok
Singapore · Tokyo · Sydney

Drug Dosage
The authors and the publisher have exerted every effort to ensure that drug selection and dosage set forth in this text are in accord with current recommendations and practice at the time of publication. However, in view of ongoing research, changes in government regulations, and the constant flow of information relating to drug therapy and drug reactions, the reader is urged to check the package insert for each drug for any change in indications and dosage and for added warnings and precautions. This is particularly important when the recommended agent is a new and/or infrequently employed drug.

Printed in Switzerland on acid-free paper by
Thür AG Offsetdruck, Pratteln
ISBN 3-8055-5740-X

Contents

Introductory Lecture

LeRoith, D.; Shemer, J.; Roberts, C.T., Jr.	Evolutionary Origins of Intercellular Communication Systems: Implications for Mammalian Biology	1

Multiple Endocrine Diseases

Scherbaum, W.A.	Introduction	7
Riley, W.J.	Autoimmune Polyglandular Syndromes	9
Calender, A.; Schuffenecker, I.; Lenoir, G.M.	The Genetics of Multiple Endocrine Neoplasia (MEN)	16
Padberg, B.C.; Holl, K.; Schröder, S.	Pathology of Multiple Endocrine Neoplasias 2A and 2B: A Review	24
Raue, F.; Zink, A.	Clinical Features of Multiple Endocrine Neoplasia Type 1 and Type 2	31

Anabolic and Metabolic Effects of Growth Hormone Action

Saenger, P.	Introduction	36
Clemmons, D.R.; Underwood, L.E.	Role of Insulin-Like Growth Factors and Growth Hormone in Reversing Catabolic States	37
Gertner, J.M.	Growth Hormone Actions on Fat Distribution and Metabolism	41
Haymond, M.W.; Horber, F.F.	The Effects of Human Growth Hormone and Prednisone on Whole Body Estimates of Protein Metabolism	44
Caprio, S.; Boulware, D.; Tamborlane, V.	Growth Hormone and Insulin Interactions	47

Intersexuality

Sizonenko, P.C.	Introduction	50
Swaab, D.F.; Gooren, L.J.G.; Hofman, M.A.	Gender and Sexual Orientation in Relation to Hypothalamic Structures	51
Hawkins, J.R.	Genetic Determinants of Testis Development in Normal and Abnormal Individuals	62
Voutilainen, R.	Differentiation of the Fetal Gonad	66
Josso, N.	Anti-Müllerian Hormone and Sertoli Cell Function	72
Hughes, I.A.; Williams, D.M.; Batch, J.A.; Patterson, M.N.	Male Pseudohermaphroditism: Clinical Management, Diagnosis and Treatment	77
Aarskog, D.	Syndromes and Genital Dysmorphology	82
	Author Index	86
	Subject Index	87

Introductory Lecture

Horm Res 1992;38(suppl 2):1–6

D. LeRoith
J. Shemer
C.T. Roberts, Jr.

Diabetes Branch, National Institute of Diabetes and Kidney and Digestive Diseases, National Institutes of Health, Bethesda, MD, USA

Evolutionary Origins of Intercellular Communication Systems: Implications for Mammalian Biology

Key Words
Endocrine
Evolution
Neurocrine
Peptide hormones

Abstract
Traditionally, the two major systems of intercellular communication (i.e. the nervous and endocrine systems) were considered separate functional and anatomical entities. Recent studies have provided evidence that the biochemical elements of these systems have common early phylogenetic origins and have suggested that, with the exception of their anatomical diversity, all the systems of intercellular communication are biochemically similar. On the basis of these findings, we suggest that the overlaps between the nervous and endocrine systems, the widespread tissue production of hormones, and other phenomena are now more easily understood.

Introduction

Systems of intercellular communication in mammals and vertebrates are very sophisticated and, at first glance, it appears that the best-studied systems (i.e. the endocrine and nervous systems) have diversified significantly. For example, classic endocrine systems discharge their signals (i.e. hormones) into the circulation, whereas the nervous system releases its signals (i.e. neurotransmitters) into a synapse. Closer analyses of the fundamental biochemical elements involved in these systems of intercellular communication reveal, however, that they are actually very similar (fig. 1). Thus, the synthesis and release of the signals, the nature of the receptor molecules on the target cell, and the post-receptor effector molecules are similar, if not identical, in these systems as well as in other types of communication systems, such as those employing paracrine, exocrine, or autocrine modes of action.

In this review, we will summarize some recent findings which suggest that the biochemical elements of intercellular communication have common early phylogenetic origins. We propose that these common origins are the basis for many biological phenomena in mammals that have heretofore not been easily explained, and indicate the importance of these findings to mammalian biology.

D. LeRoith
Diabetes Branch
National Institute of Diabetes and Kidney and Digestive Diseases, National Institute of Health
Bethesda, MD (USA)

0301–0163/92/0388–0001
$ 2.75/0

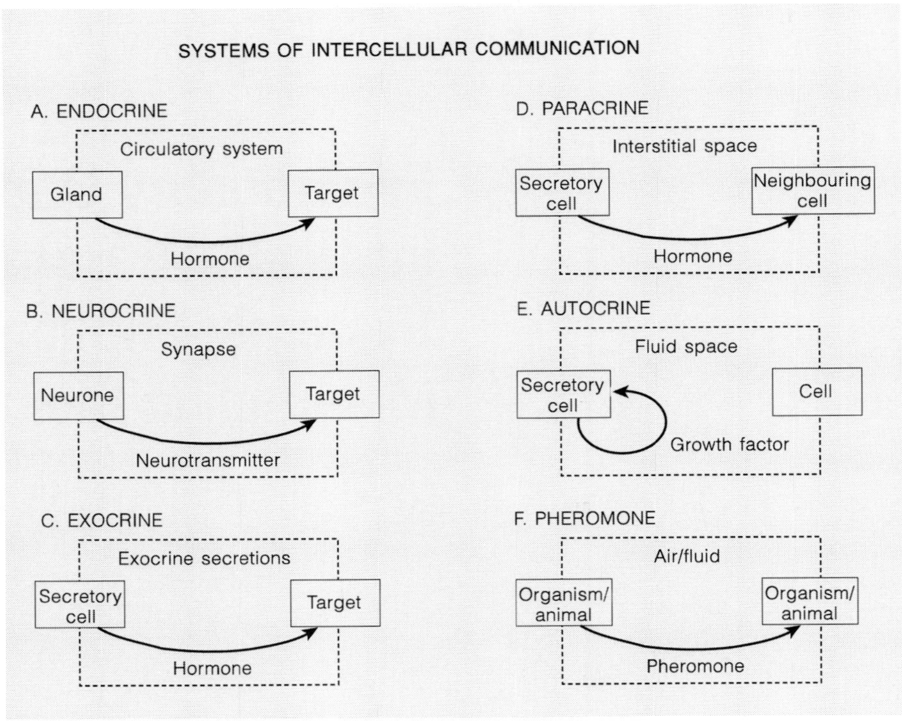

Fig. 1. Although anatomically distinct systems of intercellular communication are well-described, the biochemical elements and fundamental properties are similar. Thus, in each system, the signal molecule is synthesized and released from a particular cell or tissue and traverses an air or fluid space to reach a target cell where it interacts with a receptor to stimulate a post-receptor effector mechanism.

Peptide Hormones in Multicellular Invertebrates

A large number of vertebrate-type peptide hormones have been detected in every class of multicellular invertebrates studied. These hormones, which include insulin, glucagon, cholecystokinin and adrenocorticotrophic hormone (ACTH), have been detected using immunoassay or bioassay techniques in extracts from such diverse sources as insects, molluscs, annelids, etc. [1, 2].

Insulin-related molecules in particular have been identified in insects and molluscs [3, 4]. Insulin-related material was found in the head of the blowfly and was characterized using anti-bovine insulin antiserum (fig. 2). Interestingly, extirpation of the median neurosecretory cells, which contained the insulin-related material, resulted in the elevation of trehalose and glucose levels in the haemolymph of the blowflies (fig. 3). Replacement therapy with purified mammalian insulin or partially purified blowfly brain insulin reversed these changes, suggesting that brain insulin may control carbohydrate homoeostasis in the blowfly. The effects of insulin in mammals are mediated by insulin receptors and, in fact, cDNAs encoding an insulin receptor homologue have been isolated from *Drosophila*. Sequence analysis has revealed some similarity with mammalian insulin receptors, particularly in the conserved tyrosine kinase domain [5]. Another insulin-like molecule, prothoracicotrophic hormone, regulates metamorphosis in silkworms. Recent characterization of this regulatory brain peptide demonstrated sequence similarity of 50–60% with both insulin and insulin-like growth factor I.

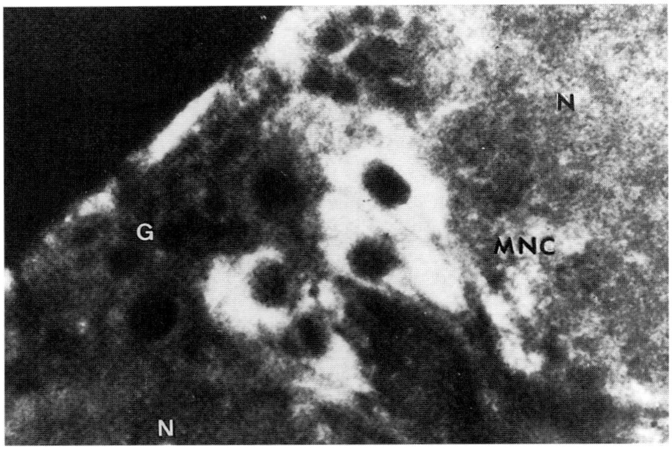

Fig. 2. Insulin immunofluorescence in cells of blowfly brain. The cells reacting with the anti-bovine insulin antiserum are the median neurosecretory cells of the pars intercerebralis. Adapted from [4].

Table 1. Microbial materials closely resembling messenger peptides of vertebrates

Hormone-related material	microbe
Insulin	*Tetrahymena* spp, *Escherichia coli*
Somatostatin	*Tetrahymena* spp, *E. coli*
ACTH	*Tetrahymena* spp, *E. coli*
Neurotensin	*E. coli,* Pseudomonas spp
TSH	*Clostridium perfringens*
hCG	Many bacteria

ACTH = Adrenocorticotrophic hormone; TSH = thyroid stimulating hormone; hCG = human chorionic gonadotrophin.

Table 2. Hormone-binding materials in microbes that resemble vertebrate-type receptors

Vertebrate hormone bound	microbe
hCG	*Pseudomonas maltophilia*
TSH	*Escherichia coli, Yersinia enterocolitica*
Opioid	*Amoeba proteus*
Corticosterone	*Candida albicans*
Oestrogen	*Saccharomyces cerevisiae*

hCG = Human chorionic gonadotrophin; TSH = thyroid stimulating hormone.

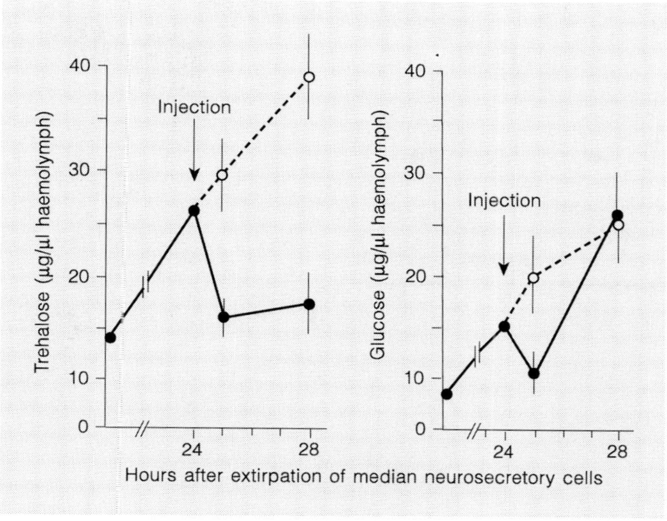

Fig. 3. Extirpation of the median neurosecretory cells (MNC) containing insulin in the blowfly brain causes an elevation of trehalose and glucose in the haemolymph. When purified insulin from mammalian sources or from blowfly brain was injected into the flies lacking MNC, a rapid but temporary fall in trehalose and glucose was achieved. Adapted from [4].

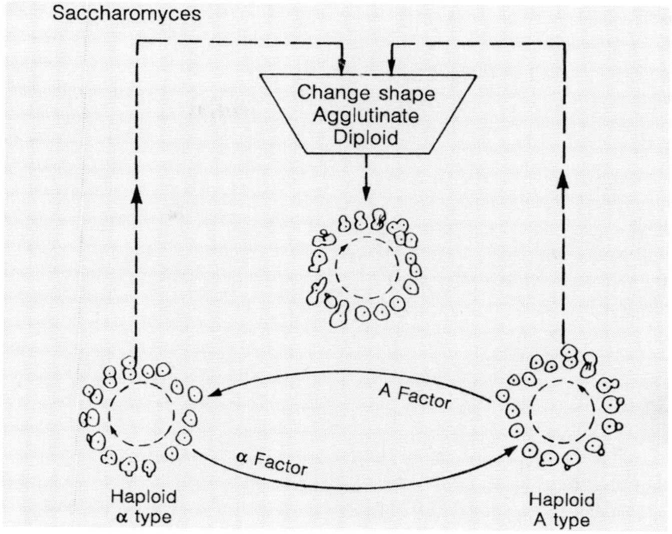

Fig. 4. Sex pheromones in *Saccharomyces cerevisiae*. The life cycle of *S. cerevisiae* involves two haploid types (α and A), as well as sporulating diploids. Each haploid produces mating pheromones that induce specific changes in the other haploid cell. This allows sexual conjugation to occur with the formation of diploid zygotes. Adapted from [6].

Thus, classic vertebrate-type peptide hormones are common in multicellular invertebrates, despite the fact that typical well-defined vertebrate endocrine glands are not found in these lower species. Interestingly, the major site of peptide hormones in non-vertebrates is the nervous system.

Vertebrate-Type Peptide Hormones in Unicellular Organisms

In extending the studies described above, we and others have found classic peptide hormones in a wide variety of unicellular organisms (table 1). Receptor-like molecules have also been demonstrated in microbes (table 2). These findings have prompted the suggestion that systems of intercellular communication similar to those in higher organisms are found at this early phylogenetic level. Indeed, unicellular organisms communicate in a manner similar to that seen in higher organisms [1, 2].

One such communication system is found in brewers' yeast, *Saccharomyces cerevisiae* (fig. 4). Interestingly, yeast α mating factor can bind, albeit with low affinity, to luteinizing hormone releasing hormone receptors in rat pituitary glands and cause the release of luteinizing hormone [6]. Furthermore, the normal receptor for α mating factor in yeast is a G-protein-related molecule with a predicted ter-

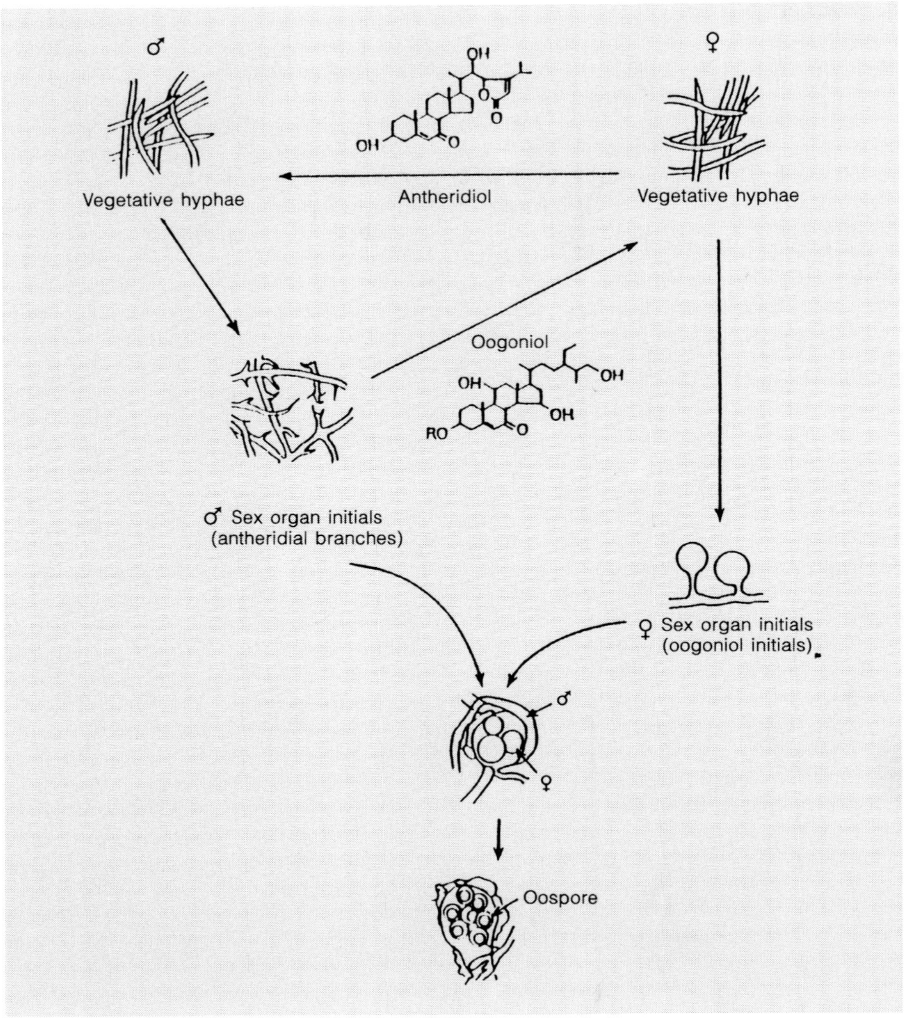

Fig. 5. Sexual pheromones and mating in the aquatic fungus *Achlya*. In *Achlya*, the female secretes the sterol pheromone antheridiol, which induces the formation of antheridiol branches and a second pheromone, oogonial in the male. The branches grow towards the female and the oogoniol causes the female to form oogoniol initials. Nuclei within each sex organ undergo meiosis, forming oospheres and sperm. Sperm pass through a fertilization tube formed between the sex organs and fuse with oospheres to produce zygotes (oospores), which germinate and produce new diploid individuals. Adapted from [7].

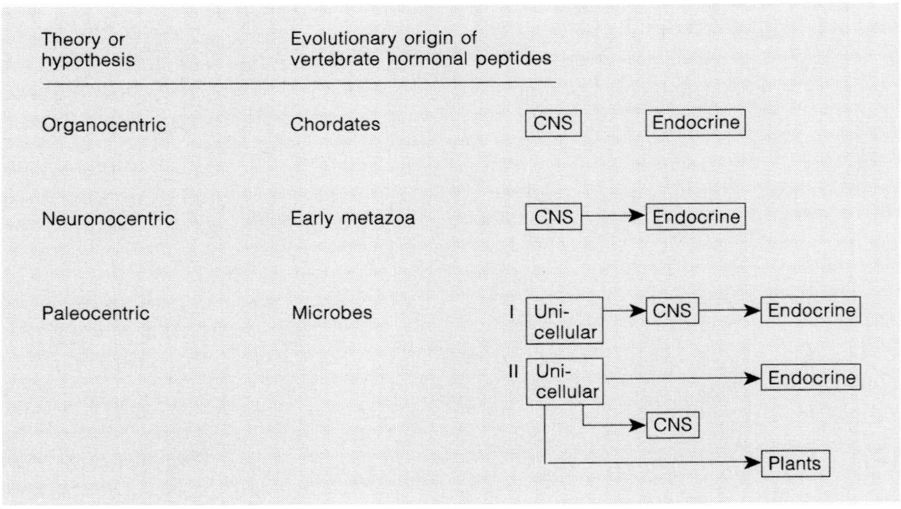

Fig. 6. Summary of theories developed to explain the origins of the nervous and endocrine systems of communication. Originally the nervous and endocrine systems were considered separate entities (organocentric). Subsequently, with the discovery of neuroactive substances in early metazoa, a theory was developed, which suggested that the nervous system of metazoa gave rise to the vertebrate endocrine system (neuronocentric). Finally, the data described in this and other reviews suggest that these major systems arose simultaneously (paleocentric) and, in addition, gave rise to similar systems in the plant kingdom.

tiary structure similar to the receptor-associated G proteins found in vertebrates. Another well-characterized system is found in the water fungus, *Achlya* [7], where male and female species communicate using steroid hormones and typical steroid receptors (fig. 5).

These findings strongly suggest that the origins of intercellular communication may have arisen at the unicellular level. If this hypothesis is correct, similar molecules should be found in plants, as the animal and plant kingdoms diverged at the level of unicellular organisms (fig. 6). Indeed, evidence for vertebrate-type peptide hormones has been found in various plants (table 3).

Table 3. Materials in higher plants that resemble messenger peptides of vertebrates [8]

Vertebrate analogue	Plant
LHRH	Oats
TRH	Alfalfa
Opioids	Wheat
Interferon	Tobacco
Insulin	Spinach
Somatostatin	Spinach, tobacco

LHRH = Luteinizing hormone releasing hormone; TRH = thyroid stimulating hormone releasing hormone.

Relevance of Early Intercellular Communication Systems to Mammalian Biology

The finding that the biochemical elements of vertebrate systems of intercellular communication have early common phylogenetic origins led us to re-examine a number of phenomena in vertebrates that were previously difficult to comprehend [9] (table 4). Traditionally, an endocrine gland was considered to be a unique source of particular hormones, and production of these hormones by non-endocrine tissues was considered 'ectopic'. As tissues throughout the animal and plant kingdoms produce similar hormones, the question of ectopic hormone production needs to be readdressed and efforts should be focused on demonstrating the regulation and function of these hormones in non-endocrine tissues.

Thus, the classic distinction between systems of intercellular communication as endocrine, neurocrine, paracrine, etc. is no longer appropriate. These common evolutionary origins suggest that, since the biochemistry is common, the artificial separation is only the result of anatomical diversity. Indeed, overlaps between nervous and endocrine systems with coexistence of neuroactive and peptide hormones in individual neurons are now readily understood [10].

Table 4. Overlaps between systems of intercellular communication

1 Hormones are synthesized by many non-endocrine tissues
2 Classic gastrointestinal hormones (e.g. cholecystokinin) are synthesized in the brain
3 Neuropeptides (e.g. somatostatin) are synthesized in non-nervous tissue
4 Tissue growth factors (e.g. nerve growth factor and insulin-like growth factor) have structural and functional similarities with classic hormones

Summary

Intercellular communication is not unique to organisms that possess anatomically well-developed nervous, endocrine, or other systems. It is an essential system in all forms of life. Recent evidence suggests that the biochemical elements of intercellular communication systems are extremely well-conserved throughout the animal and plant kingdoms.

References

1 LeRoith D, Shiloach J, Roth J: Is there an earlier phylogenetic precursor that is common to both the nervous and endocrine systems? Peptides 1982;3:211–215.

2 LeRoith D, Shiloach J, Berelowitz M, et al: Are messenger molecules in microbes the ancestors of the vertebrate hormones and tissue factors? Fed Proc 1983;42:2602–2607.

3 LeRoith D, Lesniak MA, Roth J: Insulin in insects and annelids. Diabetes 1981;30:70–76.

4 Duve H, Thorpe A, Lazarus NR: Isolation of material displaying insulin-like immunological and biological activity from the brain of the blowfly *Calliphora vomitora*. Biochem J 1979;184:221–227.

5 Petruzzelli L, Herrera R, Garcia R, et al: The insulin receptor of *Drosophila melanogaster*. Cold Spring Harbor Symp Quant Biol 1985; 3:115–122.

6 Loumaye E, Thorner J, Catt KJ: Yeast mating pheromone activates mammalian gonadotrophs: Evolutionary conservation of a reproductive hormone. Science 1982;218: 1324–1325.

7 Horgen PA: The role of the steroid sex pheromone antheridiol in controlling the development of male sex organs in the water mold, *Achlya*; in O'Day DH, Horgen PA (eds): Sexual Interactions in Eukaryote Microbes. New York, Academic Press, 1981, pp 155–178.

8 LeRoith D, Delahunty G, Wilson G-L, et al: Evolutionary aspects of the endocrine and nervous systems. Recent Prog Horm Res 1986;42: 549–587.

9 Roth J, LeRoith D, Shiloach J, et al: The evolutionary origins of hormones, neurotransmitters, and other extracellular chemical messengers. Implication for mammalian biology. N Eng J Med 1982;306:523–527.

10 LeRoith D, Shiloach J, Roth J: Coexistence of multiple neuroactive materials in individual neurons. Do recent evolutionary studies provide a rational interpretation?; in Palay VC, Palay SL (eds): Coexistence of Neuroactive Substances in Neurons. New York, John Wiley, 1984, pp 411–421.

Horm Res 1992;38(suppl 2):7–8

W.A. Scherbaum

Introduction

In this symposium we tried to provide an update on the most relevant aspects of endocrine diseases that primarily involve more than one gland. From their pathogenesis and clinical appearance two very distinct conditions were considered: polyendocrine autoimmunity and multiple endocrine neoplasia (MEN).

It is an intriguing fact that nearly every endocrine gland may be affected by an autoimmune attack which may either leave the function of the organ intact (subclinical autoimmunity) or lead to endocrine disturbances. These may result in hypo- or hyperfunction of the gland and with atrophy or hypertrophy of the tissue, depending on the specificity of the cellular and humoral autoimmunity. Why several endocrine autoimmune diseases may occur in one individual more often than by chance still remains an enigma. Genetic factors, viral triggers and common antigenic determinants on target tissues have been considered. In a balanced overview Dr Riley covers autoimmune polyglandular syndromes. Knowledge of polyendocrine syndromes enables screening programmes for associated autoantibodies and biochemical function tests to be developed which may reveal subclinical disease and allow early treatment. The most spectacular advances in the understanding of endocrine autoimmune diseases have come from analysis of the major histocompatibility complex (MHC) genes and their products, the HLA class I and HLA class II antigens. Cloning HLA class II genes and the recognition of certain polymorphisms associated with protection from or predisposition to Type 1 (insulin-dependent) diabetes mellitus has provided a new understanding of its immunopathogenesis at a molecular level.

In MEN syndromes, benign or malignant tumours occur in two or more endocrine glands in a single patient. The first description of MEN by Erdheim in 1903 was mainly based on autopsy findings. Initial reports deal with individual patients, and the familial trait of MEN was later recognized. Our present knowledge of these syndromes has enabled systematic screening to be developed in predisposed families. Recent advances in clinical recognition and biochemical detection, in the fine pathology and genetics of MEN, have provided new insights which deserve separate reviews.

Dr Padberg and his colleagues covers the pathology of MEN 2A and MEN 2B, where it focuses on the association between the morphology and the clinical characteristics of these syndromes related to their prognostic value. The pathological process is almost always multicentric, often resulting in bilateral involvement of organs. The authors review evidence to suggest that immunocytochemistry may be a valuable aid in discriminating between the different stages in the development of c-cell hyperplasia to c-cell neoplasia or from nodular hyperplasia of the adrenal medulla to phaeochromocytoma. They also discuss the difficulties in defining histological criteria which can discriminate between hyperplastic and neoplastic parathyroid proliferation and the possible means of discriminating histologically between sporadic and autosomal dominant forms of MEN.

The recognition of a tumour of the parathyroid, the endocrine pancreas, the anterior pituitary, thyroid c-cells or the adrenal medulla should alert the physician to consider MEN and to arrange for the appropriate endocrinological investigations to be carried out. Dr Raue and Dr Zink summarize the clinical findings in MEN 1 and MEN 2. They provide recommendations for screening programmes which may allow early diagnosis. Such efforts have been shown to improve the long-term outcome of these patients.

Modern methods of molecular biology have made it possible to investigate the genetic events involved in malignant proliferation and to search for inherited cancer genes.

Dr Calender and his colleagues summarize recent advances in the identification of gene carriers among the relatives of patients affected with MEN. Characterization of restriction fragment length polymorphisms of cloned DNA segments and linkage analysis as well as genomic analysis of tumour DNA are described with reference to MEN. MEN 1 and MEN 2 gene loci have recently been mapped to chromosomes 11 and 10, respectively. The safe detection of such individuals using a DNA test performed once in life would allow endocrine screening tests to be restricted to those at risk. However, there will still be uncertainty as to when the biochemical changes and clinical symptoms will develop.

I hope that these reviews will help clinicians and basic scientists to understand the pathogenesis and clinical features of polyendocrine syndromes better and to stimulate further research on these topics.

Horm Res 1992;38(suppl 2):9–15

W.J. Riley

Department of Pathology and Laboratory Medicine, University of Florida College of Medicine, J Hillis Miller Health Center, Gainsville, FL, USA

Autoimmune Polyglandular Syndromes

Key Words
Autoantibodies
Autoimmune diseases
Addison's disease
Review
Mucocutaneous candidiasis
HLA DR antigens

Abstract
Autoimmune polyglandular syndromes originally defined by Blizzard, Maclaren and Neufeld were classified into three constellations based on the clinical clustering of the various component diseases. Type I and type II are reasonably well circumscribed entities with type III being an ill-defined group. The autoimmune nature of these diseases has been based on the presence of lymphocytic infiltration in the affected gland, organ specific autoantibodies in the serum, cellular immune defects and an association with the HLA DR/DQ genes or immune response genes. Autoantibodies to the various endocrine and non-endocrine tissues not only offer a diagnostic clue to the autoimmune nature of diseases but also can be used to identify asymptomatic individuals who are at risk of developing other component diseases of the syndrome. In this review the clinical and serological spectrum of type I and II APS will be discussed.

Introduction

Over the past four decades, several disorders, which were previously thought to be idiopathic, are now considered to be autoimmune in origin. These disorders include both non-organ specific or systemic diseases (e.g. systemic lupus erythematosus) and organ specific diseases (e.g. Addison's disease, Hashimoto's thyroiditis and insulin dependent diabetes mellitus – IDDM). These autoimmune diseases share several characteristics which demonstrate that their origin is autoimmune in nature.

The affected organ is infiltrated by mononuclear cells. In 1912, Hashimoto first reported the histopathological findings of lymphocytic 'struma lymphomatosa' in several women with goitre [1]; autoimmune thyroiditis is now commonly cited as Hashimoto's thyroiditis because of his original description of the classic histopathology. Lymphocytic infiltration of the pancreatic islets is also found in IDDM and of the adrenal gland in Addison's disease [2, 3]. The role of these mononuclear cells has been extensively studied in IDDM, not only in man, but also in animal models of IDDM [4–7]. The types of mononuclear cells in these infiltrates are likely to vary, depending on the stage of the disease. Both CD4+ and CD8+ lymphocytes have each been described as the predominant cell type [5] and, importantly, these cells have been cloned in the mice model of IDDM – the NOD mouse. Transfer of the disease has been accomplished in these mice with these clones and appears to be dependent on the presence of CD4+ lymphocytes. Thus, it is likely that these characteristic cellular infiltrates reflect the effector cells of the immunological process. Unfortunately, several endocrine diseases, such as Addison's disease, have no animal model in which this hypothesis of cell-mediated immune destruction can be tested.

The presence of cellular immune defects is another characteristic of these disorders, which supports such an hypothesis. Nerup described cellular hypersensitivity to adrenal extracts in patients with Addison's disease [8, 9], and significant cellular immune defects have been described in patients with Addison's disease and chronic

W.J. Riley
Department of Pathology and Laboratory Medicine
University of Florida College of Medicine
PO Box 100275, J. Hillis Miller Health Center
Gainesville, FL (USA)

0301–0163/92/0388–0009
$ 2.75/0

mucocutaneous candidiasis [10]. We have also described a defect in the ability of CD4+CD45RO lymphocytes to provide help in a T-B lymphocyte co-culture system in IDDM [11]. This apparent paradox of impaired immune function in a disease with aggressive autoimmune destruction of an organ has always been intriguing.

Several other characteristic findings, such as the presence of organ specific autoantibodies, the common association of multiple endocrine disorders in the same patient and/or in the same family, and the association with genes in the immune response region, specifically the HLA-DR and DQ genes, have been used as evidence of an autoimmune origin for these disorders.

Table 1. Type I APS

Endocrine disorders	
Hypoparathyroidism	90%
Addison's disease	60%
Gonadal failure	45%
Autoimmune thyroid disease	10%
IDDM	1%
Hypopituitarism	
Diabetes insipidus	
Nonendocrine disorders	
Mucocutaneous candidiasis	75%
Malabsorption syndromes	25%
Alopecia	20%
Pernicious anemia	15%
Chronic active hepatitis	10%
Vitiligo	5%
Sjörgen's syndrome	
Dystrophy of nails and dental enamel	
Progressive myopathy	

Clinical Spectrum of Autoimmune Polyglandular Syndromes

Several of these endocrine diseases often occur in the same patient, which has prompted the use of the term autoimmune polyglandular syndrome (APS) [12, 13]. These endocrine diseases can be grouped into two relatively well-defined clusters and have been called type I APS (Blizzard's syndrome or autoimmune polyendocrinopathy-candidiasis-octodermal dystrophy – APECED) and type II APS (Schmidt-Carpenter's syndrome [10, 12–17]. Type I APS consists of three primary disorders – Addison's disease, hypoparathyroidism and chronic mucocutaneous candidiasis – and several commonly associated disorders, such as gonadal failure, alopecia, malabsorption, vitiligo, chronic active hepatitis and keratopathy (table 1). Type II APS also consists of three primary disorders – IDDM, Addison's disease and thyroid autoimmune diseases (table 2) –, although several other diseases, particularly atrophic gastritis/pernicious anaemia, occur more commonly than is usually recognized.

Table 2. Type II APS

Endocrine disorders	
Addison's disease	100%
Autoimmune thyroid disease	70%
IDDM	30%
Gonadal failure	10%
Hypopituitarism	<1%
Nonendocrine disorders	
Alopecia	
Pernicious anemia	
Chronic active hepatitis	
Vitiligo	
Premature greying	

Type I APS

The clinical expression of type I APS was initially documented by Neufeld et al. [12]. Recently, Perheentupa et al. found that every patient in their large cohort had at least developed chronic mucocutaneous candidiasis before the age of 30 years, most commonly in childhood, but not exclusively; they did, however, emphasize the variability of the clinical disease [15]. The disease occurs in both male and female patients, and although multiple cases have been described within one family, the disease is predominantly sporadic [12, 18].

The first disease that is recognized clinically in patients with type I APS is often detected within the first decade of life. Infants commonly present with persistent mucocutaneous candidiasis that is resistant to usual routine baby care. Eventually, the nails become involved. Although not all infants with chronic mucocutaneous candidiasis will have type I APS, a significant number will, and it is essential that the diagnosis is considered. In a recent review of patients from eight medical centres, 22 out of 43 children with chronic mucocutaneous candidiasis had developed alopecia, hypoparathyroidism or Addison's disease [19]. Ketoconazole has been effective in controlling the candidiasis in most patients. Other severe infections were the cause of death in six of these children with chronic mucocutaneous candidiasis [19]. Hypocalcaemia due to the hypoparathyroidism may present as tetany or seizures. Hypoparathyroidism was the most common endocrinopathy, which affected 80–90% of patients [12, 15]. Addison's disease usually does not present until after 6 years of age. However, a study in Finland showed that when adrenal failure occurred at an early age, the other components of the disease were less common [15], but this has not been our experience in a smaller number of patients. Gonadal failure and chronic active hepatitis usually occur after the onset of Addison's disease. Gonadal dysfunction developing after puberty is, however, common in men, but premature menopause is often seen in women [20], though we have seen several males who have progressed slowly or not at all through puberty. Intestinal malabsorption is found in at least 9% of patients and causes difficult problems in determining the appropriate dose of drugs.

During the last few years, other diseases have been recognized in these patients. One of the more devastating is the development of a progressive myopathy which can lead to the patients' demise [21]. The aetiology is unclear as no lymphocytic infiltration is found in the muscle, only focal atrophy of type 2 fibres. Sjörgen's syndrome can be debilitating, though not life threatening [12].

Type II APS

Type II APS is by far the most common form of polyendocrine failure. The syndrome occurs at all ages, but more commonly in adults. There is a strong female predominance, and other family members are often found to have diseases in the complex or autoantibodies to these organs. The initial classification of type II APS required the presence of Addison's disease and either thyroid autoimmune disease and/or IDDM [12]. Whether patients without Addison's disease, but with either IDDM, one of the thyroid autoimmune diseases or autoimmune atrophic gastritis/pernicious anaemia, should be classified as having type II APS is debatable.

The age of onset and temporal relationship of the component diseases varies much more than in type I APS [12, 17]. Thyroid autoimmune disease or IDDM is found in 50% of patients with Addison's disease, but the predominant association is with thyroid disease, as Schmidt originally described [17]. Carpenter has, however, since described the less common association of the triad, that is with IDDM [22]. Interestingly, those patients with IDDM and Addison's disease are more likely to have developed IDDM before the Addison's disease [17]. This is consistent with recent data on the risk of progression to IDDM in patients with Addison's disease who have islet cell autoantibodies (ICA). Our data and a recent report suggest that the risk is less despite the high titres of ICA [23]. In our own group of 88 patients with IDDM and hypothyroidism, hypothyroidism was diagnosed at the same time or after IDDM in 47 out of 52 patients who developed IDDM before the age of 20 years, but had been diagnosed equally before and after diagnosis of IDDM in the 33 patients who developed IDDM after 20 years of age.

The incidence of pernicious anaemia/atrophic gastritis in this complex is not fully appreciated, because the symptoms are often attributed to the primary disease. In our studies, achlorhydria after pentagastrin stimulation was found in 50% of the IDDM patients with PCA [24]. Pernicious anaemia was not found, but these patients were less than 20 years of age at the time of study. In a group of older patients with vitiligo, Betterle et al. demonstrated atrophic gastritis by biopsy in 95% of patients who were found to have PCA [25]. Thus, 95% of all patients with vitiligo will have pernicious anaemia and/or gastric atrophy. In the same study, Addison's disease and/or adrenocortical autoantibodies were also found in 2% of patients. Chronic active hepatitis and primary biliary cirrhosis have been reported to be part of the type II APS syndrome, though they are not as common as in type I APS. Vitiligo, alopecia and premature greying of the hair are relatively common, easily identified and should alert the physician to the possible presence of other diseases.

Recently, several uncommon and interesting diseases, such as hypophysitis, have been reported in association with type II APS [26–30]. Most cases of hypophysitis do not occur in type II APS, but are primarily related to pregnancy and often present between the second month of gestation and 14 months postpartum [31]. Treatment of the underlying adrenal insufficiency in this disorder has improved or resolved the impending or actual failure of the thyroid gland and ovary [32–34]. In our experience, many patients will eventually relapse despite the adrenocortical replacement. Women have been able to complete a successful pregnancy despite Addison's disease [35–38]; in one patient with oophoritis, with increased luteinizing hormone (LH) and follicle stimulating hormone (FSH) concentrations, therapy with high dose steroids allowed a successful pregnancy [36].

Immunogenetics of Type I and Type II APS

Although the incidence of type I APS is sporadic, there have been several reports of the syndrome occurring in multiple siblings [10, 39–41]. Spinner, in his study of siblings with hypoparathyroidism and Addison's disease

[39], initially suggested an autosomal recessive inheritance. Figure 1 summarizes the data from these family studies and demonstrates the lack of linkage to the HLA genes. The location of the gene for this complex and whether there are multiple genes remains to be determined. Although our study did not find an association with genes in the HLA region, one group of investigators have demonstrated an association with HLA-A28 and HLA-A3 in their Finnish patients with type I APS [16, 42, 43]. HLA-A28 was more common in patients with hypoparathyroidism and HLA-A3 in those with ovarian failure [43]. In our studies, none of the component diseases was found to be associated with a particular HLA allele.

In contrast to the above findings in type I APS, affected siblings with IDDM and/or type II APS share the same HLA-haplotypes to a marked degree. Our own studies, as well as those documented in the literature, indicate that the degree of sharing on chromosome 6 in type II APS is similar to the findings in IDDM, with 55% of sibling pairs sharing both HLA genes with their affected sibling (HLA-identical), 40% sharing one (haploidentical), and only 5% sharing neither [17, 42, 44]. Similarly, type II APS is also strongly associated with the same HLA-DR genes DR3 and DR4. In fact, more patients with type II APS are heterozygotes, having both HLA-DR3 and HLA-DR4, than patients with IDDM [42, 45]. Because of these similarities, one might assume that these diseases may also have similar HLA-DQ genes [46]. Type II APS appears to have a dominant mode of transmission, with important genes lying within the HLA genetic complex on chromosome 6, as well as others that do not.

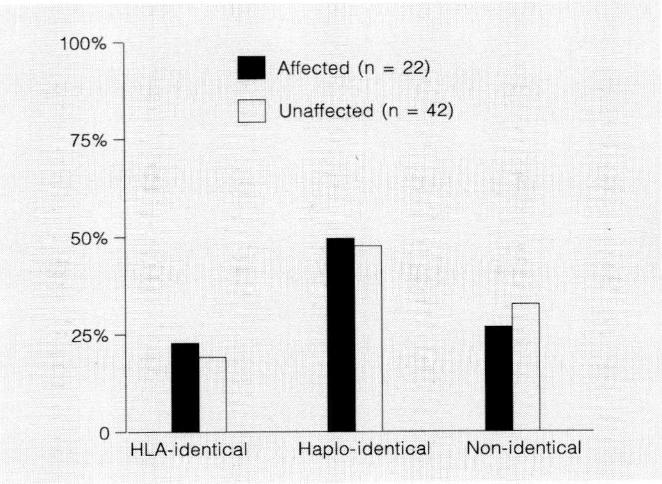

Fig. 1. Type I APS HLA-sharing in 33 siblings. Combined data from [10, 40, 41, 43].

Autoantibodies and Autoantigens in Autoimmune Polyglandular Syndrome

Adrenal Cortical Antibodies

Several types of autoantibodies against the adrenal gland have been described in patients with Addison's disease and APS. In nearly 65% of patients with autoimmune Addison's disease, autoantibodies directed against the cytoplasmic antigen are detected by indirect immunofluorescence [47]. The antigen for this autoantibody remains unknown. Differential ultracentrifugation has localized the antigen to the microsomal and plasma membrane fraction. The subcellular fractions, against which the antibody reacted, were enriched for cytochrome c reductase and 5'-nucleotidase [48]. A 55 kD protein has been identified by immunoprecipitation in this sera in 13 out of 23 patients with Addison's disease [49].

These autoantibodies have been used by several investigators to identify individuals at risk of developing autoimmune adrenal disease [20, 50–52]. Although screening the general population is of little benefit, because of a negligible prevalence in the general population, screening of patients at high risk of developing adrenal disease is quite effective. Chronic mucocutaneous candidiasis, hypoparathyroidism, vitiligo, diabetes and thyroid disease will be found in only 5–50% of these patients. As many as 50% of asymptomatic individuals with adrenal autoantibodies will develop adrenocortical insufficiency within 3–5 years. These patients will demonstrate a classical pattern of compensated hypoadrenalism with increased adrenocorticotrophic hormone (ACTH) and plasma renin activity levels prior to the loss of corticosteroid and aldosterone production. Gradually, the 24-hour production of aldosterone and cortisol will decrease until a stage of adrenal insufficiency is diagnosed. Since the adrenal insufficiency can be fatal if left untreated, monitoring of these patients with adrenal antibodies is important and should be recommended.

Adrenal autoantibodies have also been detected by methods other than indirect immunofluorescence. The development of a radioimmunoassay or enzyme-linked immunosorbent assay (ELISA) for the detection of adrenal autoantibodies makes screening more feasible [53, 54]. In addition, surface reactive antibodies have been detected in the sera of patients with Addison's disease. More recently, antibodies that block the ACTH stimulation on adrenocortical cells have been detected [55]. In the accompanying grafts, immunoglobulins were extracted by protein G separation and used in a tissue culture system with a Y1 murine adrenocortical cell line. This cell line responds to ACTH by the production of the second message, cyclic AMP. Figure 2 shows a dose-dependent decrease in the production of cyclic AMP with increasing concentrations of immunoglobulins in 3 out of 4 patients with Addison's disease. In the control subject and 1 patient with Addison's disease, this had little to no effect on cyclic AMP production. Thus, blocking antibodies appear to exist in Addison's disease, similar to those seen in Hashimoto's thyroiditis.

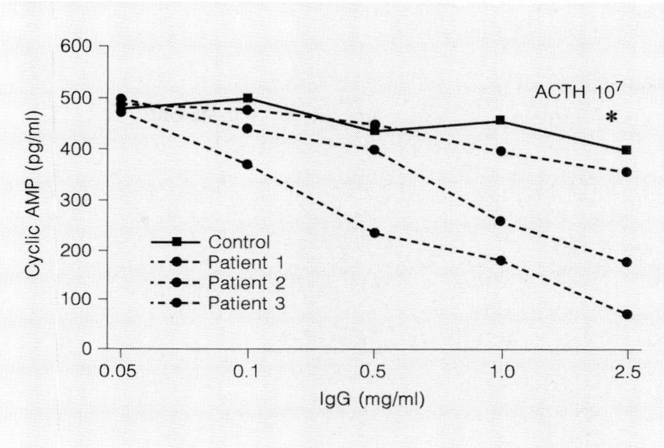

Fig. 2. Inhibition of cyclic AMP response to ACTH in Addison's disease.

Steroidal Cell Antibodies

Patients with autoimmunity to their gonadal tissue often show reactivity against the various sex steroid-secreting tissues, such as the placental syncytiotrophoblast, luteal cells in the ovary, and the Leydig cells in the testes [56]. One of the unique features of the autoantibodies is the specificity of steroid-producing cells and the lack of organ specificity; sera from female patients will not only react to the luteal cells in the ovarian tissue, but also to the Leydig cells of the testes. Thus, these autoantibodies differ from the other endocrine autoantibodies. It is likely that the antigen against which these antibodies are directed, is an enzyme common in all steroid-producing tissues.

More recently, Moncayo developed an ELISA for the detection of autoantibodies against the LH-human chorionic gonadotrophin (HCG) receptor and the hormone receptor complex in 13 out of 30 patients with ovarian failure. A constant and recurring feature in many of these autoimmune diseases is, therefore, the number of autoantibodies against not only antigens in the cytoplasm, but also several surface antigens including hormone receptors.

Parathyroid Antibodies

Parathyroid antibodies were originally described by Blizzard et al. in 1966 [57]. Few laboratories have, however, been able to duplicate these specific autoantibodies and, recently, many groups have suggested that the autoantibodies detected by indirect immunofluorescence using parathyroid tissue are actually mitochondrial antibodies. Parathyroid gland is known to be a good source of mitochondria and, thus, the reactivity would not be unexpected [58]. Brandi has recently studied sera from patients with autoimmune hypoparathyroidism using a complement-dependent cytotoxicity assay. IgM autoantibodies were detected in the sera of patients with hypoparathyroidism [59], which appeared to be directed against the parathyroid endothelium [60].

Cardiac Autoantibodies

Recently a group from the Middlesex Hospital described the presence of autoantibodies against cardiac muscle in patients with type I APS [61]. They suggest that these autoantibodies are related to the increased risk of hypertension, since 28 out of 166 patients with hypertension have autoantibodies to the cardiac muscle. This is quite an interesting and unique finding, which needs to be verified by other groups, and poses yet another problem for these patients.

References

1 Hashimoto H: Zur Kenntnis der lymphomatösen Veränderung der Schilddrüse (struma lymphomatos). Arch Klin Chir 1912;97:219–248.
2 Gepts W: Islet morphology in type I diabetes. Behring Inst Mit 1984;39–41.
3 Spinner MW, Blizzard RM, Gibbs J, et al: Familial distributions of organ specific antibodies in the blood of patients with Addison's disease and hypoparathyroidism and their relatives. Clin Exp Immunol 1969;5:461–468.
4 Boitard C, Yasunami R, Dardenne M, Bach JF: T cell-mediated inhibition of the transfer of autoimmune diabetes in NOD mice. J Exp Med 1989;169:1669–1680.
5 Weber CJ, Zabinski S, Koschitzky T, et al: The role of CD4+ helper T cells in the destruction of microencapsulated islet xenografts in nod mice. Transplantation 1990;49:396–404.
6 Hutchings PR, Simpson E, O'Reilly LA, et al: The involvement of Ly2+ T cells in beta cell destruction. J Autoimmun 1990;3:101–109.
7 Robertson RP, Seaquist ER, Walseth TF: G proteins and modulation of insulin secretion. Diabetes 1991;40:1–6.
8 Nerup J, Andersen V, Bendixen G: Anti-adrenal cellular hypersensitivity in Addison's disease. IV. In vivo and in vitro investigations on the mitochondrial fraction. Clin Exp Immunol 1970;6:733–739
9 Nerup J, Bendixen G: Anti-adrenal hypersensitivity in Addison's disease. II. Correlation with clinical and serological findings. Clin Exp Immunol 1969;5:341–353.
10 Arulantham K, Dwyer JM, Genel M: Evidence for defective immunoregulation in the syndrome of familial candidiasis endocrinopathy. N Engl J Med 1979;300:164–168.
11 Schatz DA, Riley WJ, Maclaren NK, et al: Defective inducer T-cell function before the onset of insulin-dependent diabetes mellitus. J Autoimmun 1991;4:125–136.
12 Neufed M, Maclaren NK, Blizzard RM: Autoimmune polyglandular syndromes. Pediatr Ann 1980;9(4):43–53.
13 Neufeld M, Maclaren NK, Blizzard RM: Two types of autoimmune Addison's disease associated with different polyglandular autoimmune (PGA) syndromes. Medicine 1981;60: 355–362.
14 Schmidt MB: Eine biglandulare Erkankung (Nebennieren und Schilddrüse) bei Morbus addisonsii. Verh Dtsch Ges Pathol 1926;21: 212–220.
15 Ahonen P, Myllarniemi S, Sipila I, et al: Clinical variation of autoimmune polyendocrinopathy-candidiasis-ectodermal dystrophy (APECED) in a series of 68 patients. N Engl J Med 1990;322:1829–1836.
16 Ahonen P: Autoimmune polyendocrinopathy-candidosis-ectodermal dystrophy (APECD): Autosomal recessive inheritance. Clin Genet 1985;27:535–542.
17 Papadopoulos KI, Hallengren B: Polyglandular autoimmune syndrome type II in patients with idiopathic Addison's disease. Acta Endocrinol 1990;122:472–478.
18 Van Vliet E, Roep BO, Meulenbroek L, et al: Human T cell clones with specificity for insulinoma cell antigens. Eur J Immunol 1989;19: 213–216.
19 Herrod HG: Chronic mucocutaneous candidiasis in childhood and complications of non-candida infection: A report of the Pediatric Immunodeficiency Collaborative Study Group. J Pediatr 1990;116:377–382.
20 Ahonen P, Miettinen A, Perheentupa J: Adrenal and steroidal cell antibodies in patients with autoimmune polyglandular disease type I and risk of adrenocortical and ovarian failure. J Clin Endocrinol Metab 1987;64:494–500.
21 Bech K, Hier Madsen M, Feldt Rasmussen U, et al: Thyroid function and autoimmune manifestations in insulin-dependent diabetes mellitus during and after pregnancy. Acta Endocrinol 1991;124:534–539.
22 Carpenter CCJ, Solomon N, Silverberg S, et al: Schmidt's syndrome (thyroid and adrenal insufficiency): A review of the literature and a report of 15 new cases including ten instances of coexistent diabetes mellitus. Medicine 1964;43:153–180.
23 Bosi E, Becker F, Bonifacio E, et al: Progression of type I diabetes in autoimmune endocrine patients with islet cell antibodies. Diabetes 1991;40:977–984.
24 Riley WJ, Toskes PP, Maclaren NK, et al: Predictive value of gastric parietal cell autoantibodies as a marker for gastric and hematologic abnormalities associated with insulin-dependent diabetes. Diabetes 1982;31:1051–1055.
25 Betterle C, Caretto A, De Zio A, et al: Incidence and significance of organ-specific autoimmune disorders (clinical, latent or only autoantibodies) in patients with vitiligo. Dermatologica 1985;171:419–423.
26 Barkan AL, Kelch RP, Marshall JC: Isolated gonadotrope failure in the polyglandular autoimmune syndrome. N Engl J Med 1985;312: 1535–1540.
27 Pestell RG, Best JD, Alford FP: Lymphocytic hypophysitis. The clinical spectrum of the disorder and evidence for an autoimmune pathogenesis. Clin Endocrinol 1990;33: 457–466.
28 Arvanitakis C, Knouss RF: Selective hypopituitarism. Impaired cell-mediated immunity and chronic mucocutaneous candidiasis. JAMA 1973;225:1492–1495.
29 Pouplard A: Pituitary autoimmunity. Horm Res 1982;16:289–297.
30 Cappuccio FP, Markandu ND, Buckley MG, et al: Raised plasma levels of atrial natriuretic peptides in Addison's disease. J Endocrinol Invest 1989;12:205–207.
31 Cosman F, Kalmon DP, Holub DA: Lymphocytic hypophysitis. Report of 3 new cases and review of literature. Medicine 1989;68: 240–256.
32 Burrows AW: Reversible hypothyroidism after steroid replacement for Addison's disease. Postgrad Med J 1981;57:368–370.
33 Candrina R, Giustina G: Addison's disease and corticosteroid-reversible hypothyroidism. J Endocrinol Invest 1987;10:523–526.
34 Ismail AA, Burr WA, Walker PL: Acute changes in serum thyrotrophin in treated Addison's disease. Clin Endocrinol 1989;30: 225–230.
35 Finer N, Fogelman I, Bottazzo GF: Pregnancy in a woman with premature ovarian failure. Postgrad Med J 1985;61:1079–1080.
36 Cowchock FS, McCabe JL, Montgomery BB: Pregnancy after corticosteroid administration in premature ovarian failure (polyglandular endocrinopathy syndrome). Am J Obstet Gynecol 1988;158:118–119.
37 Rabinowe SL: Immunopathogenesis and therapy of gonadal disorders and infertility; in Eisenbarth GS (ed): Immunotherapy of Diabetes and Selected Autoimmune Diseases. Boca Raton, CRC Press, 1991, pp 151–162.
38 Albert E, Dalaker K, Jorde R, et al: Addison's disease and pregnancy. Acta Obstet Gynecol Scand 1989;68:185–187.
39 Spinner MW, Blizzard RM, Childs B: Clinical and genetic heterogeneity in idiopathic Addison's disease and hypoparathyroidism. J Clin Endocrinol Metab 1968;28:795–802.
40 Kaffe S, Petigrow CS, Cahill LT, et al: Variable cell-mediated immune defects in a family with 'candida endocrinopathy syndrome'. Exp Clin Immunogenet 1975;20:397–403.
41 Wirfalt A: Genetic heterogeneity in autoimmune polyglandular failure. Acta Med Scand 1981;210:7–13.
42 Maclaren NK, Riley WJ: Inherited susceptibility to autoimmune Addison's disease is linked to human leukocyte antigens-DR3 and/or DR4, except when associated with type I autoimmune polyglandular syndrome. J Clin Endocrinol Metab 1986;62:455–459.
43 Ahonen P, Koskimies S, Lokki ML, et al: The expression of autoimmune polyglandular disease type I appears associated with several HLA-A antigens but not with HLA-DR. J Clin Endocrinol Metab 1988;66:1152–1157.
44 Eisenbarth GS, Wilson PW, Ward F, et al: The polyglandular failure syndrome: Disease inheritance, HLA type and immune function. Ann Intern Med 1979;91:528–533.
45 Latinne D, Vandeput Y, De Bruyère M, et al: Addison's disease: Immunological aspects. Tissue Antigens 1987;30:23–24.
46 Morel PA, Dorman JS, Todd JA, et al: Aspartic acid at position 57 of the HLA-DQ beta chain protects against type I diabetes: A family study. Proc Natl Acad Sci USA 1988;85: 8111–8115.

47 Nerup J, Lindholm J, Soborg M, et al: Organ-specific antibodies in idiopathic panhypopituitarism, primary thyroid and adrenal insufficiency. Acta Med Scand 1969;185:293–296.
48 Bright GM, Singh I: Adrenal autoantibodies bind to adrenal subcellular fractions enriched in cytochrome-c reductase and 5'-nucleotidase. J Clin Endocrinol Metab 1990;70:95–99.
49 Furmaniak J, Talbot D, Reinwein D, et al: Immunoprecipitation of human adrenal microsomal antigen. FEBS Lett 1988;231:25–28.
50 Ketchum CH, Riley WJ, Maclaren NK: Adrenal dysfunction in asymptomatic patients with adrenocortical autoantibodies. J Clin Endocrinol Metab 1984;58:1166–1170.
51 Guérin V, Bene MC, Amiel C, et al: Decreased lymphocyte function-associated antigen-1 molecule expression on peripheral blood lymphocytes from patients with Graves' disease. J Clin Endocrinol Metab 1989;69:648–653.
52 Riley WJ, Maclaren NK, Neufeld M: Adrenal autoantibodies and Addison disease in insulin-dependent diabetes mellitus. J Pediatr 1980;97:191–195.
53 Kosowicz J, Gryczynska M, Bottazzo GF: A radioimmunoassay for the detection of adrenal autoantibodies. Clin Exp Immunol 1986;63:671–679.
54 Stechemesser E, Scherbaum WA, Grossmann T, et al: An ELISA method for the detection of autoantibodies to adrenal cortex. J Immunol Methods 1985;80:67–76.
55 Wulffraat NM, Drexhage HA, Bottazzo GF, et al: Immunoglobulins of patients with idiopathic Addison's disease block the in vitro action of adrenocorticotropin. J Clin Endocrinol Metab 1989;69:231–238.
56 Elder ME, Maclaren NK, Riley WJ: Gonadal autoantibodies in patients with hypogonadism and/or Addison's disease. J Clin Endocrinol Metab 1981;52:1137–1142.
57 Blizzard RM, Chee D, Davis W: The incidence of parathyroid and other antibodies in sera of patients with idiopathic hypoparathyroidism. Clin Exp Immunol 1966;1:119–128.
58 Betterle C, Caretto A, Zeviani M, et al: Demonstration and characterization of anti-human mitochondria autoantibodies in idiopathic hypoparathyroidism and in other conditions. Clin Exp Immunol 1985;62:353–360.
59 Brandi ML, Aurbach GD, Fattorossi A, et al: Antibodies cytotoxic to bovine parathyroid cells in autoimmune hypoparathyroidism. Proc Natl Acad Sci USA 1986;83:8366–8369.
60 Fattorossi A, Aurbach GD, Sakaguchi K, et al: Anti-endothelial cell antibodies: Detection and characterization in sera from patients with autoimmune hypoparathyroidism. Proc Natl Acad Sci USA 1988;85:4015–4019.
61 Caforio AL, Wagner R, Gill JS, et al: Organ-specific cardiac antibodies: Serological markers for systemic hypertension in autoimmune polyendocrinopathy. Lancet 1991;337:1111–1115.

Horm Res 1992;38(suppl 2):16–23

A. Calender
I. Schuffenecker
G.M. Lenoir

Laboratory of Genetics,
Edouard Herriot Hospital, Lyon, France

The Genetics of Multiple Endocrine Neoplasia (MEN)

Key Words
Multiple endocrine neoplasia
Genetics
Gene
Predictive screening

Abstract
Multiple Endocrine Neoplasia (MEN) refers to the family of diseases characterized by hyperplasia and/or tumoral proliferation in various organs derived from the neural crest. MEN are transmitted in an autosomal dominant fashion in affected pedigrees with a high degree of penetrance. MEN 1 and MEN 2A/B loci have recently been mapped, respectively, to chromosomes 11 and 10 by linkage analysis using polymorphic DNA markers. These discoveries will lead (1) to a rapid understanding of the physiopathological pathway determining such syndromes and (2) to major clinical impact through the genetic screening.

Introduction

Recent progress in genetics and molecular biology has increased our understanding of the mechanisms of susceptibility to inherited diseases, including familial forms of cancer. Inherited cancers are thought to result from at least two mutational events. The first is germinal and confers the inherited predisposition to the individual, the second, somatic mutation, is acquired and leads to the development of cancer [1]. In non-hereditary cases, both events occur post-zygotically in somatic cells. Occasionally, dominant mutations (usually deletions), leading to inherited cancers, are detectable by cytogenetic examination. However, in the majority of cases, the hereditary nature of the cancer or proliferative disease is inferred from inspection of the patient's pedigree or from some unusual feature of the clinical presentation. For instance, the presence of a predisposing genetic trait in a family member, a large number of cancers transmitted in a Mendelian pattern, the presence of bilateral tumours in childhood, or the association of a cancer and particular congenital malformations may signal an underlying mutation predisposing to a malignant disease [2].

The appearance of multiple tumours in a family might also be explained by exposure to a common environmental hazard or genetic susceptibility to a mutagenic factor. Harmful aspects of the environment have been estimated to cause 70% of cancers, but their importance is yet to be evaluated in the case of inherited syndromes or cancer with familial aggregation.

Molecular biology has opened the way to characterizing mutant genes that cause abnormal growth and confer genetic susceptibility to cancers. This is particularly true for the multiple endocrine neoplasia (MEN) syndromes, in which tumours of two or more endocrine glands occur in the same individual [3]. Progress in hormone assays and in the recognition of clinical disorders associated with excessive hormone production have facilitated early diagnosis and management of patients. Nevertheless, major problems remain in the preclinical evaluation of the disease, before the major complications associated with the adenomas observed in MEN occur. All forms of MEN seem to be inherited as autosomal dominant traits [3], as established by the identification of a large number of pedigrees. This report summarizes recent discoveries in the genetics of MEN 1 and MEN 2 syndromes, in terms of the identification of gene carriers in the relatives of affected patients. If it were possible to identify carriers of the gene by a simple DNA test, biochemical and endocrine screening efforts could concentrate on those at risk. Genetic risk prediction

A. Calender
Laboratory of Genetics
Edouard Herriot Hospital
Place d'Arsonval, F–69437 Lyon Cedex (France)

has an impact on better screening and earlier diagnosis in MEN families. It also represents a major step in the identification of the genes involved in diseases and in understanding the pathogenesis of these endocrine tumour syndromes.

Methodological Aspects of Genetic Mapping and its Use for Screening

The investigation of the genetic events involved in malignant proliferation and the search for inherited cancer genes have become possible in the past few years as a result of advances in molecular biology. Cloned human DNA sequences are now available, corresponding to defined genes and also to non-coding DNA segments, some of them showing sequence polymorphism. The latter have been used as molecular probes in linkage studies and to increase the sensitivity of cytogenetic investigations using tumour biopsies.

Restriction Fragment Length Polymorphism

A large number of cloned DNA segments have been localized on the human genome, and for some, restriction fragment length polymorphisms (RFLPs) have been characterized [4]. RFLPs are the result of variations in the primary DNA sequence of individuals, which may be caused by single base changes, deletions, nucleotide additions, segment translocations or the presence of repetitive sequences. These polymorphisms, occurring frequently in non-coding regions, may lead to the presence or absence of a cleavage site for restriction enzymes, which cleave the DNA in a sequence-specific manner. Using standard protocols, the total genomic DNA obtained from a few millilitres of blood is hybridized following restriction enzyme digestion with defined polymorphic probes selected around the disease locus. For each RFLP the exact number and size of alleles will vary in the population with known frequency, in relation to the number of recognition sites for the restriction enzyme. RFLPs have to be directly related to the natural allelic variation which occurs between individuals at a genetic locus and are critical for linkage analysis.

Linkage Analysis

RFLPs represent good genetic markers for linkage studies in families and for localizing a disease susceptibility gene. RFLPs are inherited in a Mendelian manner and their inheritance can be followed, together with the disease in an affected pedigree [5]. A RFLP allele co-segregates with the disease if the two genetic loci are close together on the chromosome. Genes that are far apart do not consistently co-segregate and show recombination because of crossing-over during meiosis. The recombination fraction θ (θ is the number of recombinants divided by the total number of offspring resulting from informative meioses) varies from 0 (in the case of closely adjacent genes) to 0.5 (when the genes are far apart and localized on different chromosomes). The probability that the two loci are genetically linked is expressed by the LOD-score, defined as the log of the odds ratio favouring linkage [6] (the odds ratio favouring linkage represents the likelihood that the two loci are linked for a specified recombination value, versus the likelihood that the two loci are not linked). LOD-scores are usually evaluated over a range of θ, to ascertain the genetic distance and the maximum probability favouring linkage between the two loci. For each RFLP, defined superior and inferior limits of the LOD-score permit evaluation of the degree of linkage with the disease locus. A LOD-score of +3 indicates a probability in favour of linkage of 1000 to 1. A LOD-score of –2 indicates a probability against linkage of 100 to 1 and is taken to exclude linkage between two genetic loci. Computer programs are available to calculate such parameters from genetic data obtained from pedigrees [7], and also enable the results from different families to be combined.

Tumour Genomic DNA Analysis

Analysis with RFLP probes may identify differences between the tumour DNA and the normal tissue genomic DNA from a patient. Such heterogeneity reflects loss of specific DNA segments or chromosomal regions; designated as loss of alleles or loss of heterozygosity [8] (fig. 1). Molecular analysis of tumour DNA has to be related to cytogenetic observations. The finding of a consistent region of chromosomal loss in tumour cells indicates a likely chromosomal location of a suppressor gene. These observations demonstrate that complementary cytogenetic and molecular investigations on tumour material would greatly facilitate studies into the search for inherited cancer genes.

Genetic Screening of Endocrine Tumour Syndromes

The two major forms of MEN are referred to as type 1 and 2. MEN 1, or Wermer's syndrome, is characterized by the combined occurrence of hyperplasia or tumours of the parathyroid glands, the pancreatic islet cells and the anterior pituitary gland [3, 9] (table 1). MEN 2 is characterized by the occurrence of medullary thyroid carcinoma (MTC), in association with phaeochromocytoma. Variants of this syndrome are: MEN 2a, MTC-only, and MEN 2b. MEN 2a, or Sipple's syndrome, is the most common form, in which development of MTC is associated with phaeochromocytoma and parathyroid hyperplasia. In MTC-only, MTC seems to be the only manifestation of the syndrome [3]. In MEN 2b, or Gorlin's syndrome, parathyroid involvement is absent, and affected patients present with a marfanoid appearance, neuromas of the buccal cavity and visceral ganglioneuromatosis. In MEN 2, screening through DNA linkage analysis, in addition to the conventional screening programme used for affected families, is of great value in the clinical management of the syndrome.

Linkage Analysis for MEN 2

Clinical Aspects. MEN 2 is a dominantly inherited cancer syndrome, but clinical penetrance is incomplete. In MEN 2a, the lifetime penetrance of medullary thyroid cancer is greater than 80%. In families where it appears, the penetrance of phaeochromocytoma is approximately 50%. Parathyroid hyperplasia may be observed in 10–40% of cases [10]. Because thyroid C cell proliferation is the major manifestation of MEN 2a, calcitonin measurements made before and after a stimulus by pentagastrin represent the most useful screening test for detecting the first signs of the disease and the gene carriers. If the pentagastrin stimulation test is positive, the penetrance is almost complete, and 90% of gene carriers can be detected before they are 25 years of age [11]. Families with a history of MTC are identified in France through a national registry established by the Groupe d'Etude des Tumeurs à Calcitonine (GETC) [12]. Thirty-four families have now been studied with a subset of 24 families with origins in France. Diagnosis of MEN 2a was made when at least two first-degree relatives were documented with a MTC, either by pentagastrin stimulation or by histological analysis. Individuals with MTC were screened for phaeochromocytoma with a urinary dose of vanillylmandelic acid and catecholamines. In 14 families, MTC segregates alone; this is defined as the MTC-only inherited syndrome. These well-characterized pedigrees were subjected to genetic linkage analysis.

Linkage Analysis with Polymorphic DNA Probes. The gene for MEN 2a has been mapped to chromosome 10, close to the retinol-binding-gene-protein locus (hRBP) in the pericentromeric region [13, 14]. A set of polymorphic DNA markers is available to allow preclinical and early carrier diagnosis. The accuracy of DNA-based prediction is increased by using all the probes closely linked together and flanking the MEN 2a gene. Previous studies have demonstrated that the use of only one informative marker, such as hRBP, may allow more precise prediction of the carrier state than the use of the pentagastrin stimulation test alone, although there is still a 2–4% prediction error [15]. The association of a DNA assay with two closely linked probes, and the pentagastrin-stimulated calcitonin assay significantly increases the accuracy of the risk evaluation [16]. The availability of up to 10 polymorphic markers flanking the MEN 2a locus will further reduce the residual uncer-

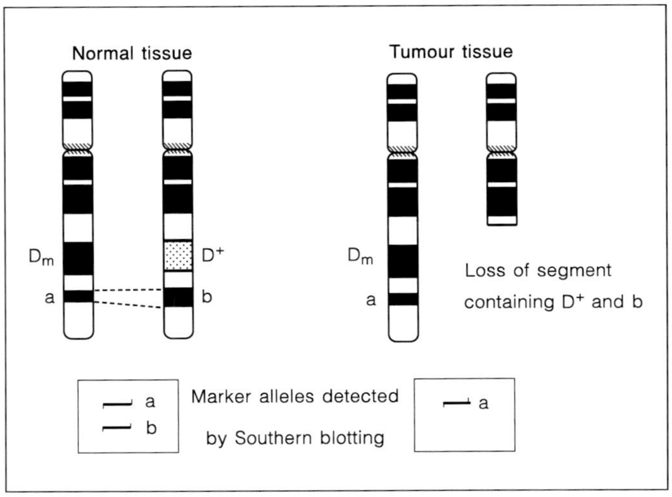

Fig. 1. Detection of chromosomal loss in tumours by Southern blotting. A pair of chromosomes is shown from the normal tissue and the tumour tissue of the same patient. D_m is a germ-line recessive mutation which predisposes to disease. D^+ is the normal allele of the same gene. Mutation causing loss of the remaining normal allele at this locus in a somatic cell leads to tumour formation. a and b are two alleles of a DNA sequence polymorphism (RFLP) which provide genetic markers. Loss of marker allele b in tumour biopsies indicates the somatic mutational event which has also led to loss of the remaining normal allele D^+ at the disease locus (adapted from Thakker and Ponder [3]).

Table 1. Main tumour targets in MEN 1

Endocrine glands	Cases, %
Parathyroid	90
Endocrine pancreas	80
Pituitary	65
Adrenal cortex	35
Thyroid (epithelial)	20
Carcinoid tumours	10–20

tainty in DNA-based predictions. Extensive genetic analysis of a large number of MEN 2 families allows the construction of a linkage map of the pericentromeric region of chromosome 10 [16]. Five of these markers (TB14–34, D10s34, MEN203, D10s94 and D10Z1) show no recombination with the MEN 2a locus. A maximum LOD-score of 30.5 was obtained at a distance of 0 centimorgan from the MEN 2a locus to the MEN203 and D10s94 markers. Multipoint linkage analysis performed with MEN203-D10s94-hRBP estimates the linked fraction of families to be 80–100% [Narod et al., in preparation]. It is important to note that 1 centimorgan corresponds to 1 megabase pair, therefore the distance between the markers and the morbid locus might still be great at the physical level. Nevertheless, the availability of polymorphic probes showing 0% recombination with the MEN 2a locus represents a step forward in the search for the gene.

Genetic Homogeneity of MEN 2 Syndromes. Both MEN 2a and MTC-only families are linked to the same polymorphic markers in the pericentromeric region of chromosome 10 [17, 18]. These probes were also recently demonstrated to be informative in MEN 2b [19]. Among 90 families with hereditary MTC, consisting of 51 families with MEN 2a, 19 families with MTC-only and 20 families with MEN 2b, there has not yet been a report of an unlinked family. Hereditary MTC is believed to be sufficiently genetically homogeneous for the purpose of genetic counselling [Narod et al., in preparation]. The authors suggest that the three presentations of hereditary MTC represent allelic mutations of the same locus with variable phenotypic expression. The alternative hypothesis is that the expression of a single MEN 2a mutation may vary within an extended family, leading to phenotypic heterogeneity and variations in penetrance. The two mechanisms have to be considered in the pathogenesis of MEN 2.

All recent studies suggest that the risk of phaeochromocytoma occurring in MTC-only families is low but significant [17]. Among 35 families with MTC, statistical evidence supports the hypothesis that the risk of phaeochromocytoma occurring varies in a continuous range. The division of families into those with a low penetrance and those with a high penetrance for adrenocortical tumour was favoured over the conventional classification of MTC-only and MEN 2a syndromes. The identification of adrenal tumour carriers in large pedigrees initially defined as MTC-only families suggests that the limits between MTC-only and MEN 2a inherited syndromes have to be re-evaluated. These phenotypic variants are probably manifestations of different alleles of the same gene, or result from two tightly linked mutations.

Considered together, the data fit the model of different subgroups of MTC families with various penetrances for phaeochromocytoma in affected carriers over 20 years of age. The possibility that other genes, or environmental factors, may affect the penetrance of adrenal tumours among carriers cannot be discounted. Haplotype analysis, using the set of informative DNA markers on a large number of MEN 2 families, suggests genetic homogeneity of this syndrome [Narod et al., in preparation]. In some families, the genetic homogeneity observed around the MEN 2a locus contrasts with the phenotypic variation in the clinical course of the disease. Phaeochromocytoma appears as a clinical marker of the severity of the illness, related to the penetrance of the MEN 2a mutation. Inherited MTC without phaeochromocytoma is associated with a later age of tumour onset and a more favourable prognosis. It has been suggested that more than 50% of MEN 2b cases, which is a much more aggressive syndrome, have been caused by new mutations at the MEN 2a locus [18]. These data remain to be confirmed, but they favour the hypothesis that the three presentations of MEN 2 may account for allelic variations of the same morbid locus.

Clinical Applications. An advantage of the DNA test is its simplicity. The test need only be performed once. The age at testing remains to be evaluated in each family. Limitations of DNA analysis are that DNA should be available from two or more affected family members to determine which allele of the marker is inherited with the MEN 2 locus. The determination of risk also requires knowledge of: the mode of disease transmission (autosomal dominant in MEN); the penetrance of the disease (which remains to be better defined in the case of phaeochromocytoma); the incidence of various phenotypes; and for linkage analysis: the recombination fraction; the proportion of linked families with each marker, and the distribution of disease and marker alleles in the general population [20]. Error in any of these estimates may result in biased risk evaluation.

We consider that DNA analysis should be introduced into the screening programme for MEN 2 families. In view of the potential clinical implications of genetic prediction, an integrated protocol of biochemical and DNA screening is warranted for the time being. The results of the DNA test have to be considered in relation to the wide variation in ages at which tumours develop in hereditary MTC (fig. 2). A positive DNA test with an informative probe has to be confirmed by molecular analysis with closely linked markers. If the patient is a gene carrier, a decision must be made regarding when and how often to use calcitonin screening. When there is conversion in the pentagastrin test, surgery has to be considered as an effective treatment of the tumour. A negative DNA result leaves the individual with a residual carrier risk of 1% or less. Follow-up by pentagastrin-stimulated calcitonin screening does not seem necessary or can be carried out every 5 years [16]. In family members where the probes reveal no information, conventional follow-up must continue until conversion indicates the affected patients. Genetic screening of a large number of pedigrees and retrospective studies on the clinical course of the disease represent the best way to define the screening interval for calcitonin assay and detect preclinical lesions, before irreversible disease occurs. In conclusion, the availability of several polymorphic markers close to the MEN 2 locus introduces the possibility of presymptomatic diagnosis, preclinical surgical management of MTC and prevention of phaeochromocytoma. Haplotype analysis remains useful for mapping the gene, and the residual uncertainty in DNA prediction will be removed as soon as the MEN 2 gene has been cloned and the intragenic mutations have been identified.

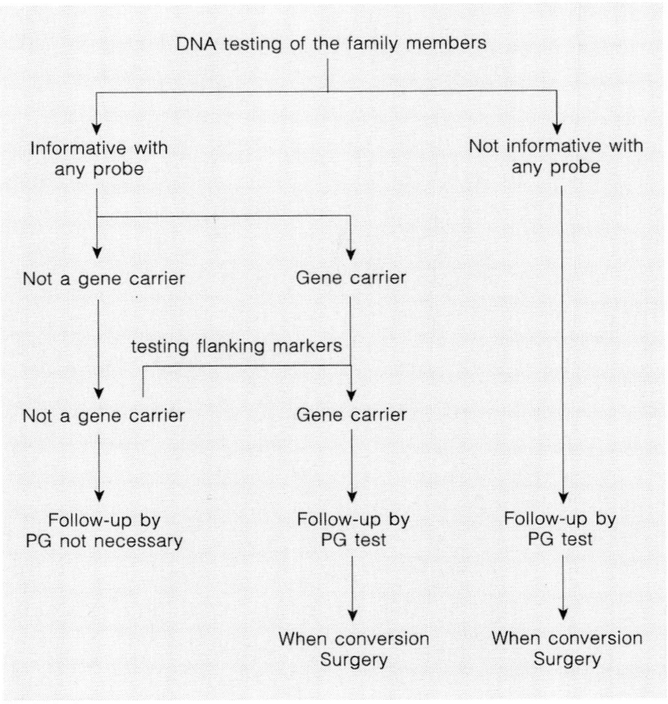

Fig. 2. A general screening protocol in the case of a familial history of MEN 2a (at least two cases). Testing family members with one or two informative probes indicates the potential gene carriers. Such individuals have to be tested further with flanking markers to confirm the DNA testing. Follow-up by pentagastrin-stimulated calcitonin assay (PG test) is necessary to assess preclinical lesions in gene carriers and to make other therapeutic decisions.

Linkage Analysis for MEN 1

Clinical Aspects. Patients with MEN 1 are characterized by the occurrence of hyperplasia or malignant tumours of the parathyroid glands, the pancreatic islet cells and the anterior pituitary gland, and in some cases associated tumours, such as carcinoid and thyroid epithelial proliferation [9]. It was initially proposed that these tumours, occurring in different endocrine tissues, had a common neuroectodermal origin, within cells of the amine precursor uptake decarboxylation system. However, the relationship between MEN 1 and the APUD system remains to be defined, considering the particular cytochemical characteristics of parathyroid cells [3]. The diversity of anatomical lesions in MEN 1 suggests a genetic heterogeneity or complex patterns of intragenic mutations in the MEN 1 locus. The incidence of the syndrome has been estimated to be 0.25% [10] and penetrance is high; 80% of patients have presented by the fifth decade. The clinical manifestations of MEN 1 are related to the sites of the tumours and to their secretion products. The clinical course of the disease is dependent on the potential complications associated with hormone hypersecretion, such as hypercalcaemia, recurrent peptic ulceration, hypoglycaemic symptoms and prolactin or growth hormone hypersecretion syndromes.

Chromosomal Localization of the MEN 1 Gene. Cytogenetic and molecular analysis of genomic DNA, in normal and tumour tissue from the same individual, showed that the pathogenesis of pancreatic as well as parathyroid lesions involves unmasking a probably recessive mutation on the long arm of chromosome 11, at band 11q13 [21, 22]. The demonstration of allele losses in MEN 1 associated tumours is in agreement with the two-mutational model postulated by Knudson [1]. Linkage studies using a set of polymorphic probes from chromosome 11 have confirmed the genetic localization of MEN 1 [23]. A peak LOD-score was obtained with the human muscle phosphorylase gene (PYGM) genetic locus, involved in McArdle's syndrome (glycogen storage disorder type IV), localized to the pericentromeric region of the long arm of chromosome 11, at band 11q13. Extended studies of DNA sequence loss in MEN 1 associated tumours, using the set of polymorphic markers, indicate that the MEN 1 locus is telomeric to PYGM in a 5 centimorgan region surrounding this marker [23]. Recently, 17 new polymorphic probes have been mapped within the 11q12–13 region and the gene order determined by physical mapping and linkage data [24]. The DNA markers linked to the MEN 1 locus provide an accu-

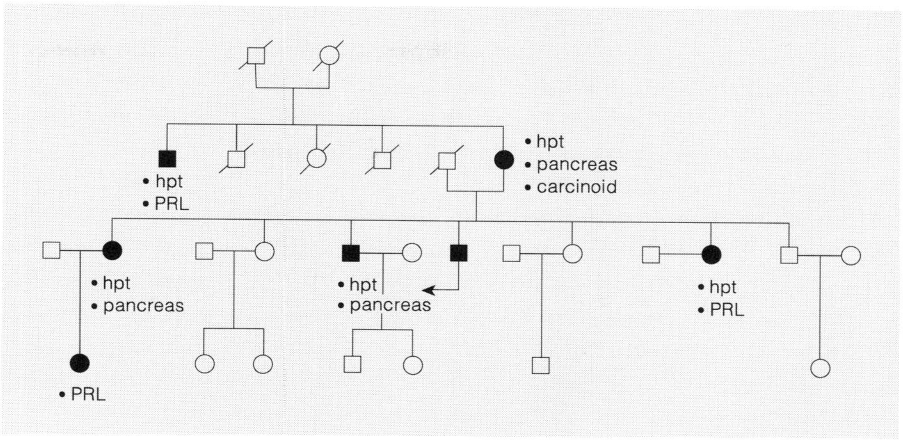

Fig. 3. An example of a pedigree with aggregation of MEN 1 cases. This family was collected through collaboration with Prof. Riou (Edouard Herriot Hospital, Lyon, France). The most common lesions observed in this family are primary hyperparathyroidism (hpt), pancreatic tumours (pancreas), prolactinoma (PRL) and in one case a carcinoid tumour.

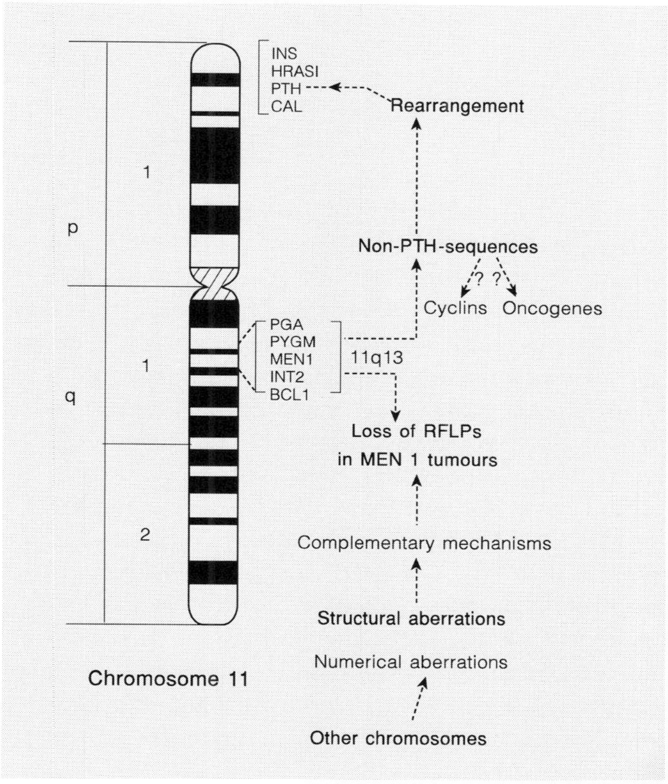

Fig. 4. Partial map of human chromosome 11 showing the locations of some genes encoding hormones, polymorphic DNA probes, oncogenes and disease loci. Chromosome 11 with Giemsa bands is schematically represented, and the probe and disease loci are shown juxtaposed to their regional localization, which has been ascertained by in situ hybridization, somatic cell hybrid or multipoint linkage studies. Two regions are represented. First, around the parathyroid hormone gene (PTH): insulin (INS), harvey RAS sarcoma 1 viral oncogene (HRAS1), and calcitonin (CAL). Second, close to the MEN 1 locus: pepsinogen (PGA), phosphorylase glycogen muscle, or McArdle syndrome glycogen storage disease type V (PYGM), murine mammary tumour virus integration site oncogene homologue (INT2), and B cell lymphoma 1 (BCL1). In some MEN 1 tumours, non-PTH sequences localized to band 11q13 are rearranged into the coding portion of the PTH gene on the short arm of the chromosome. Potential functions encoded by these non-PTH sequences are shown. Loss of RFLPs is frequently observed in MEN 1 associated insulinoma and parathyroid adenoma at band 11q13, but structural and numerical aberrations involving other chromosomes might represent complementary mechanisms in the genesis of these endocrine syndromes (adapted from Thakker and Ponder [3]).

rate set of markers which may allow premorbid identification of gene carriers.

DNA-Based Prediction of Gene Carriers. A set of highly polymorphic probes is now available close to the MEN 1 locus, with no cross-overs in a large set of families [Larsson, personal communication]. The calculated predictive accuracy with three such informative markers was estimated to be greater than 99.5%, thus demonstrating that genetic linkage analysis can be used for informed genetic counselling in MEN 1 families. Presymptomatic diagnosis of carrier patients is useful for preventing the major complications associated with hormone hypersecretion and avoiding unnecessary biochemical or radiological screening tests on non-carriers. Approximately 16 pedigrees from France were collected in our laboratory through a French collaborative network. Preliminary genetic analysis confirms linkage with the PYGM locus. An example of a MEN 1 family is shown in figure 3. The availability of a large number of probes mapped around the morbid locus will soon allow direct clinical application. As for MEN 2, haplotyping of several markers will significantly increase the information content of linkage analysis.

The Lesson of Deletion Mapping and Cytogenetic Studies. Loss of alleles was initially demonstrated in MEN 1 associated insulinoma and parathyroid tumours [21, 22]. Deletion mapping studies in sporadic primary hyperparathyroidism demonstrate that gene deletions spanning the MEN 1 locus characterize sporadic as well as MEN 1 associated parathyroid lesions, suggesting a common pathogenesis. However, loss of chromosome 11 alleles in band 11q13 is relatively infrequent in sporadic pituitary adenomas, indicating a different pathogenesis, or variations in mutational events at the MEN 1 locus, or different genes. To address this question, a collection of pituitary adenomas and other tumours from MEN 1 cases is required. Correlations between chromosomal abnormalities and functional genes on chromosome 11 have been made. As a significant example, structural abnormalities within the organization of the parathormone (PTH) gene, localized on the short arm of chromosome 11, have been identified in non-MEN 1 parathyroid adenomas, involving a sequence rearrangement and insertion of new DNA sequences [25]. Investigation of these extra-gene DNA sequences revealed it to be highly conserved in the human and mouse genome. In situ hybridization studies have localized these sequences to the long arm of chromosome 11, at band 11q13, close to the MEN 1 locus. The role of this clonal DNA rearrangement involving the PTH gene and sequences surrounding the MEN 1 locus requires further study, but suggests striking mechanisms in the genesis of sporadic as well as MEN 1 associated parathyroid tumours. Recent reports suggest that these rearranged DNA sequences contain oncogenes and functional genes, such as those coding for cyclin proteins involved in cell cycle regulation [26] (fig. 4).

Other striking observations indicate that MEN 1 pathogenesis might be more complex. Cytogenetic investigations demonstrate that some of the individuals affected with MEN 1 had an increased level of chromosome breakage compared with healthy controls [27]. Chromosome instability was found in cultured lymphocytes and fibroblasts derived from skin biopsies, with numerical and structural alterations involving mainly chromosomes 7, 12 and 18 and never chromosome 11.

Prospects. The availability of highly polymorphic probes close to the MEN 1 locus on chromosome 11 allows genetic linkage testing for genetic counselling in affected pedigrees and for the exclusion of non-gene carriers. Precise localization and further characterization of the disease gene should be supported by additional familial linkage analysis and deletion mapping studies on tumour material. Both the RFLP and cytogenetic approaches suggest that the wild-type allele of the MEN 1 gene, which is lost or altered in MEN 1 associated endocrine tumours, regulates the normal differentiation of parathyroid glands and endocrine pancreas. They also suggest that the MEN 1 predisposition would be a constitutional mutation in heterozygous form, inherited as an autosomal dominant trait. Tumour formation involves a second mutational event, a point mutation, deletion or rearrangement with a loss of heterozygosity at the same locus, leading to disease. The role of additional chromosomal abnormalities involving complementary mechanisms in tumour pathogenesis remains to be defined. Cloning the MEN 1 gene will open the way to an understanding of the genetic predisposition and the pathophysiological pathways leading to abnormal cell proliferation in distinct endocrine tissues.

Conclusions

Genetic mapping of MEN syndromes has a major clinical impact because using genetic screening allows the identification of gene carriers in predisposed families. These discoveries are also a critical step in understanding the physiological pathway determining not only these syndromes, but sporadic tumour pathogenesis in general. Typing with DNA markers is now possible, and further characterization of the disease genes will allow a precise and accurate evaluation of genetic predisposition through the analysis of intragenic mutations. For all these reasons, MEN are important models for the study of inherited cancer syndromes.

References

1 Knudson AG, Strong LC, Anderson DE: Hereditary and cancer in man; in Steinberg AG, Bearn AG (eds): Progress in Medical Genetics. New York, Grune and Stratton, 1973, vol 9, p 113.

2 Narod SA, Stiller C, Lenoir GM: An estimate of the heritable fraction of childhood cancer. Br J Cancer 1991;63:993.

3 Thakker RV, Ponder BAJ: Multiple endocrine neoplasia. Baillière's Clin Endocrinol Metabol 1988;2:1031.

4 Cooper DN, Schmidtcke I: DNA restriction fragment length polymorphisms and heterozygosity in the human genome. Human Genet 1984;66:1.

5 Wiggs J, Nordenskjöld M, Yandell D, et al: Prediction of the risk of hereditary retinoblastoma: Using DNA polymorphisms within the retinoblastoma gene. N Engl J Med 1988;318: 151.

6 Ott J: Estimation of the recombination fraction in human pedigrees: Efficient computations of the likelihood for human linkage studies. Am J Human Genet 1974;26:588.

7 Lathrop GM, Lalovel JM: Easy calculations of lod scores and genetics risks on small computers. Am J Human Genet 1984;36:460.

8 Ponder BAJ: Gene losses in human tumors. Nature 1988;335:400.

9 Wermer P: Genetic aspects of adenomatosis of endocrine glands. Am J Med 1954;16:363.

10 Lips CJM, Vasen HFA, Lamers CBHW: Multiple endocrine neoplasia syndromes. CRC Crit Rev Oncol/Haematol 1984;2:117.

11 Gagel RF, Tashjian AH, Cummings T, et al: The clinical outcome of prospective screening for multiple endocrine neoplasia type 2a. N Engl J Med 1988;318:478.

12 Calmettes C: Création d'un Groupe d'Etude des Tumeurs à Calcitonine. Bull Cancer 1984; 71:266.

13 Simpson NE, Kidd KK, Goodfellow PJ, et al: Assignment of multiple endocrine neoplasia type 2a to chromosome 10 by linkage. Nature 1987;328:528.

14 Nakamura Y, Mathew CG, Sobol H, et al: Linked markers flanking the gene for multiple endocrine neoplasia type 2A. Genomics 1989; 5:199.

15 Sobol H, Narod SA, Nakamura Y, et al: The screening for multiple endocrine neoplasia type 2A by DNA polymorphism analysis. N Engl J Med 1989;321:996.

16 Mathew CGP, Easton DF, Nakamura Y, et al: Presymptomatic screening for multiple endocrine neoplasia type 2A with linked DNA markers. Lancet 1991;337:7.

17 Narod SA, Sobol H, Nakamura Y, et al: Linkage analysis of hereditary thyroid carcinoma with and without pheochromocytoma. Human Genet 1989;83:353.

18 Norum RA, Lafrenière RG, O'Neal LW, et al: Linkage of the multiple endocrine neoplasia type 2B gene (MEN2B) to chromosome 10 markers linked to MEN2A. Genomics 1990; 8:313.

19 Lairmore TC, Howe JR, Komte JA, et al: Familial medullary thyroid carinoma and multiple endocrine neoplasia type 28 map to the same region of chromosome 10 as multiple endocrine neoplasia type 2A. Genomics 1991; 9:181.

20 Narod SA: Counselling under genetic heterogeneity: A practical approach. Clin Genet 1991; 39:125.

21 Larsson C, Skogseid B, Öberg K, et al: Multiple endocrine neoplasia type 1 gene maps to chromosome 11 and is lost in insulinoma. Nature 1988;332:85.

22 Thakker RV, Bouloux P, Wooding C, et al: Association of parathyroid tumors in multiple endocrine neoplasia type 1 with loss of alleles on chromosome 11. N Engl J Med 1989;321: 218.

23 Bystrom C, Larsson C, Blomberg C, et al: Localization of the MEN 1 to a small region within chromosome 11q13 by deletion mapping in tumors. Proc Natl Acad Sci USA 1990;87: 1968.

24 Julien C, Nakamura Y, Lathrop M, et al: A detailed genetic map of the long arm of chromosome 11. Genomics 1990;7:335.

25 Arnold A, Staunton CE, Kim HG, Gaz RD, Kronenberg HM: Monoclonality and abnormal parathyroid hormone genes in parathyroid adenomas. N Engl J Med 1988;318:658.

26 Motokuma T, Bloom T, Kim HG, et al: A novel cyclin encoded by a bel 1 linked candidate oncogene. Nature 1991;350:512.

27 Scappaticci S, Maraschio P, Del Ciotto N, et al: Chromosome abnormalities in lymphocytes and fibroblasts of subjects with multiple endocrine neoplasia type 1. Cancer Genet Cytogenet 1991;52:85.

Horm Res 1992;38(suppl 2):24–30

Pathology of Multiple Endocrine Neoplasias 2A and 2B: A Review

B.C. Padberg
K. Holl
S. Schröder

Institute of Pathology,
University of Hamburg, Germany

Key Words
Multiple endocrine neoplasia (MEN)
Medullary thyroid carcinoma
Adrenal phaeochromocytoma
Parathyroid hyperplasia
Mucosal ganglioneuromatosis

Abstract
This review describes recent findings on the morphology, function and prognosis of lesions associated with the MEN 2 syndromes. Special emphasis is placed on the analogies and discrepancies between the hereditary and nonhereditary manifestations of the endocrine proliferations involved.

Introduction

Multiple endocrine neoplasia (MEN) designates a group of autosomal-dominant hereditary syndromes that are characterized by a definite combination of hyperplasia and/or neoplastic proliferations of more than one endocrine organ. MEN 2A (Sipple's syndrome) comprises an association of C-cell hyperplasia (CCH) and medullary thyroid carcinoma (MTC) which is often bilateral, adrenal phaeochromocytoma (PCC) which is often bilateral and accompanied by adrenomedullary hyperplasia, and chief cell hyperplasia of the parathyroid glands. The morphological and functional similarity of chief cell hyperplasia of the parathyroid glands with the parathyroid changes in MEN 1 constitutes an overlap between the MEN 2A and MEN 1 syndromes (Wermer's syndrome, in combination with usually benign tumours of the endocrine pancreas and the adenohypophysis). In addition to MTC and adrenal PCC, MEN 2B (Gorlin's syndrome) includes a mucosal ganglioneuromatosis and a marfanoid appearance, but there is no evidence of parathyroid involvement [1]. The incidence of the different lesions associated with the MEN 2A and MEN 2B syndromes is listed in table 1. The morphological and clinical characteristics of, and the prognosis for these diseases (as opposed to their nonhereditary counterparts) are discussed individually below.

Medullary Thyroid Carcinoma

Medullary (C-cell) thyroid carcinoma accounts for about 10% of all types of thyroid cancer in most studies [2]; in approximately 20% of cases of MTC, the tumour occurs in the setting of MEN 2 in syndromatic association with extrathyroidal neoplasms. Conversely, more than 90% of patients with MEN 2 syndromes develop MTC, which, in most cases, represents the initial symptom of the disease [1–3]. There are no differences between hereditary and nonhereditary MTC regarding histological (predominant cell type, architecture, amyloid content), immunocytochemical (expression of polypeptides) and DNA cytophotometrical parameters [4–6]. It is, therefore, difficult to establish whether an individual case is hereditary or nonhereditary. Moreover, the prognosis in both types of MTC is determined by the same parameters (i.e. age, size of the primary tumour, lymph node metastasis) [5, 7]. Whether the identification of CCH in the thyroid adjacent to MTC is possibly a distinguishing factor, as suggested by the WHO [8], must be re-examined.

Bilateral CCH was first described by Wolfe et al. [9] as an obligatory precursor lesion of hereditary MTC. They suggested that CCH proceeds after the initial hypertrophy of individual C-cells, as a continuous process, from focal via diffuse to nodular hyperplasia. Once the basement mem-

Prof. Dr. S. Schröder
Institute of Pathology
University of Hamburg (UKE)
Martinistrasse 52, D-W-2000 Hamburg 20 (Germany)

0301–0163/92/0388–0024
$ 2.75/0

Table 1. Incidence of neoplasias associated with the MEN 2A and 2B syndromes

Neoplasia	MEN 2A, %	MEN 2B, %
Medullary thyroid carcinoma	>90	>90
Adrenal phaeochromocytoma	5–50	50
Parathyroid hyperplasia	20–100	0
Mucosal ganglioneuromatosis	0	<100

brane is breached and the interstitial stroma is invaded, nodular hyperplasia gradually changes into micro-invasive MTC [10]. Focal and diffuse CCH are defined as eccentric and circular intrafollicular proliferations of C-cells, respectively, displacing the follicular epithelium centrally in the follicle. Nodular CCH, the most advanced change in this process, is characterized by complete replacement of the thyrocytes in individual follicles by proliferating C-cells, thus resulting in solid clusters that consist entirely of parafollicular cells (fig. 1). Immunocytochemical studies promise to be valuable aids in discriminating between the different stages in the development from CCH to C-cell neoplasia: in thyroid tissues of MEN 2 patients, CEA immunocytochemistry only showed positive staining in CCH already accompanied by invasive MTC [11], while only micro-invasive MTC, and not noninvasive CCH, was reported to be histaminase-positive [12].

According to Wolfe et al. [13], the thyroid tissue bordering MTC associated with MEN 2 usually contains residues of diffuse or nodular CCH which has not yet been neoplastically transformed, while CCH is generally lacking in nonhereditary MTC. In contrast, however, several authors have described CCH in nonhereditary MTC [14–16], and 25% of patients with hereditary MTC were reported to lack accompanying CCH [16]. Furthermore, nodular CCH can occasionally also be detected adjacent to benign and malignant follicle cell tumours of the thyroid [17] and in Hashimoto's thyroiditis [18, 19]; C-cell nodules with the appearance of nodular CCH are supposed to represent a normal finding in otherwise disease-free thyroids of old patients [20]. Interestingly, in such 'physiological' non-MEN 2 associated nodular CCH, provocative testing may even result in plasma calcitonin being elevated to pathological levels [21]. Thus, the differential diagnostic value of CCH can not be regarded as reliable, and requires checking using immunocytochemical investigations including the above-mentioned antigens. In this context, it has to be noted that, with regard to the strictly bilateral occurrence of CCH in MEN 2 patients, more than 90% of hereditary MTCs present simultaneously as bilateral neoplasms [7], yet up to 30% of nonhereditary MTCs can become manifest bilaterally as well [4].

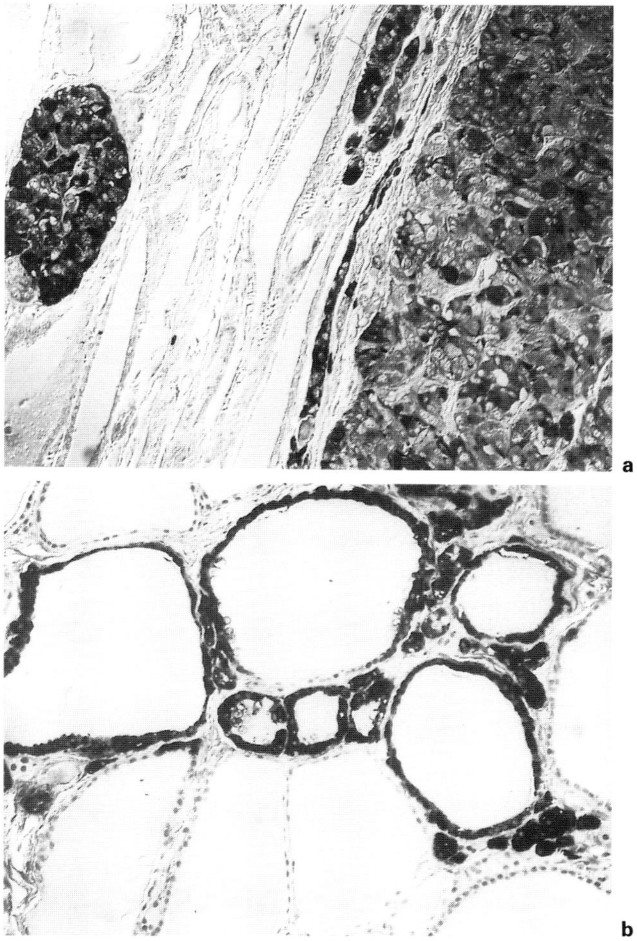

Fig. 1. C-cell hyperplasia (CCH). Nodular CCH adjacent to hereditary medullary thyroid carcinoma (right margin) (**a**). Diffuse CCH found in a tumour-free thyroidectomy specimen from a 68-year-old patient with advanced prostatic carcinoma and cervical lymph node metastases (**b**) (from [68]). Calcitonin immunostaining, 180:1.

Several investigators have shown that, compared with nonhereditary MTC, C-cell carcinomas associated with MEN 2A have a better prognosis, while neoplasms associated with MEN 2B have a far more unfavourable outcome (fig. 2) [22–25]. Since the aggressiveness of MTC generally increases with age [5, 7], Samaan et al. [26] proposed that the more favourable prognosis of MTC associated with MEN 2A merely reflected the lower mean age of such patients at diagnosis. This assumption seems implausible, however, as, according to Kakudo et al. [27], the mean age of MEN 2B patients at diagnosis (23 years) is 10 years younger than that in MEN 2A patients (38 years), and in non-hereditary MTC the mean age at diagnosis is 49 years. Thus, it seems that the differences in the malignant potential of MTC occurring as a part of the MEN 2A and 2B syndromes are genetically determined, which justifies early thyroidectomy, particularly in MEN 2B patients, as soon as elevated calcitonin levels are obtained in provocative tests [23] or, as suggested by Thompson [28], even prior to the detection of pathological hormone responses if the phenotype typical of MEN 2B is recognized.

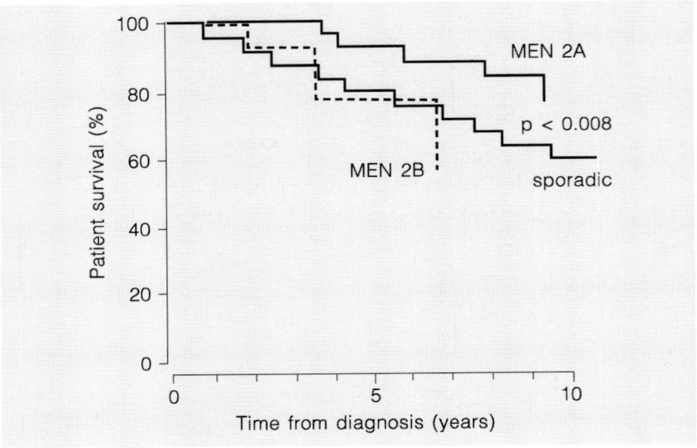

Fig. 2. Kaplan-Meier survival curves of 600 patients included in the registry of the German Medullary Thyroid Cancer Study Group (from [22]).

Adrenal Phaeochromocytoma

The incidence of adrenal PCC in patients with MEN 2A varies considerably between 5 and 50% in different studies, depending on which endocrine changes the respective investigations are focused. Most authors, however, agree that the incidence of adrenal PCC in MEN 2B is approximately 50% [2]. In the vast majority of patients, MTC is diagnosed up to two decades earlier than PCC, since PCC is found in less than 20% of patients before the age of 20 and increases in incidence with age [3]. In rare cases, PCC will precede MTC [29].

In hereditary PCC, adrenomedullary hyperplasia has been described by several authors as a morphologically defined obligatory preneoplastic lesion [30, 31]. A continuous sequence can be found from diffuse via nodular hyperplasia to PCC. The diagnosis of diffuse adrenomedullary hyperplasia can be made planimetrically with a corticomedullary ratio of less than 10:1 (the ratio in normal adrenal glands is above 10:1) and no nodules present (fig. 3) [31, 32]. Circumscribed nodules of less than 1 cm in diameter are termed nodular hyperplasia, whereas PCC is defined as a nodule larger than 1 cm [30]. Most patients with MEN 2 show adrenomedullary hyperplasia bilaterally (mostly simultaneously, but occasionally also metachronously), which is analogous to the findings in hereditary MTC (unpublished results of Carney, cited from [33]). This will naturally result in bilateral adrenal PCC, which has been described by several investigators in 70–100% of MEN 2 patients [4, 30, 34].

Apart from adrenomedullary neoplasms, the term paraganglioma has been extended in many studies to include extra-adrenal (aortico-sympathetic and visceral autonomous) paragangliomas. Such a simplified approach seems questionable, since adrenal and extra-adrenal sympathetic paragangliomas/PCC exhibit distinct clinical and biological differences, even though they are histogenetically, histo-

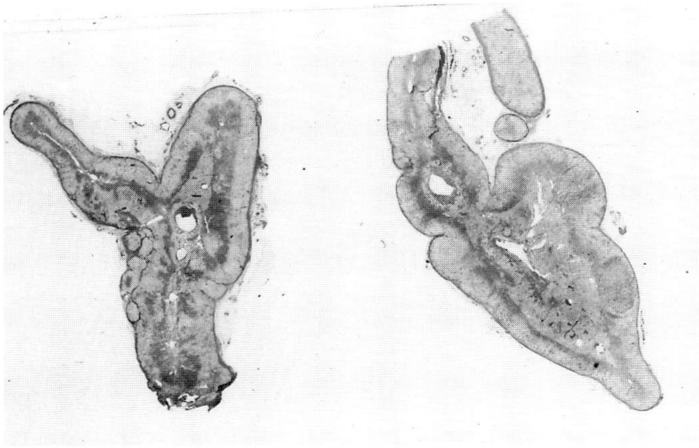

a

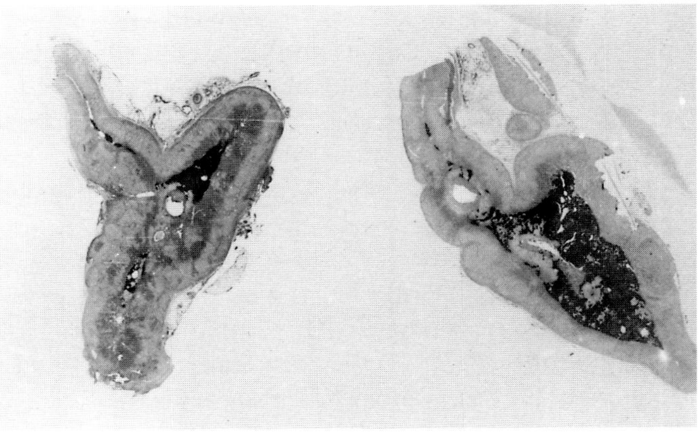

b

Fig. 3. Adrenomedullary hyperplasia. Representative cut surfaces of a normal adrenal gland (left side) and a case of adrenomedullary hyperplasia (right hand side). H&E staining (**a**) and immunocytochemistry for chromogranin A (each ×2.5) (**b**) (from [68]). To diagnose diffuse adrenomedullary hyperplasia, planimetrical determination of medullary volume performed on the whole adrenalectomy specimen cut into eight or more slides is required (for details see [49]).

structurally and functionally largely identical. In our opinion, it is highly doubtful whether extra-adrenal paragangliomas, whose incidence in association with the MEN 2 syndrome is quoted in several reviews as 10–15% [1], should be considered a part of the MEN 2 syndrome at all.

The overall malignancy rate of sympathetic PCC/paragangliomas amounts to approximately 10% [35]; in the special situation of adrenal PCC, however, lower figures have to be assumed. Thus, in the studies by van Heerden [36] and Scott and Halter [37], a malignant course was observed in 13 out of 27 extra-adrenal paragangliomas (48%), but in only 11 out of 135 adrenal PCC (8%), while in a group of 64 patients with adrenal PCC studied by Stenström et al. [38], all tumours were benign.

There have been several case reports of malignant adrenal PCC in association with MEN 2 syndrome [39]. It has been documented in a total of 7 out of 83 (8%) cases, but there has been considerable variation in the results of different studies [36, 38, 40–43]. Thus, it seems that nonhereditary and hereditary PCC associated with MEN 2 do not differ markedly in malignancy rate. The same holds true for the extremely rare combination of adrenal and extra-adrenal paragangliomas diagnosed at the same time or coincidentally in patients with nonhereditary or hereditary PCC [44, 45]. While the rate of PCC in accessory adrenal glands is undoubtedly increased in MEN 2 [46], there is no indication that there is proliferation of extra-adrenal chromaffin tissues, comparable to adrenomedullary hyperplasia, or even an increased rate of extra-adrenal paragangliomas. Thus, an extramedullary tumour was not found in any of the 83 patients with MEN 2 and PCC reported in the above studies.

Two groups, so far, have described morphological approaches to discriminate between nonhereditary PCC and PCC associated with MEN 2. Webb et al. [33], in a study of 69 cases of nonhereditary PCC, found that all exhibited a unilateral localization with residues of normal non-hyperplastic medulla at their periphery, and 93% grew as solitary unifocal tumours. Lloyd et al. [47] reported a higher density of S100-positive sustentacular cells in adrenomedullary hyperplasia and PCC associated with MEN 2, compared with that seen in nonhereditary PCC. This disagrees with our observations in a comprehensive series of 65 PCCs, in which 3 out of 20 PCCs associated with MEN 2 were entirely devoid of S100-positive sustentacular cells, whereas 12 out of 39 benign nonhereditary PCCs contained dense infiltrates of sustentacular cells [48]. Webb et al. [33] claimed sporadic (nonhereditary) PCC to grow unilaterally and to be accompanied by normal (non-hyperplastic) adrenomedullary tissue. In contrast, other authors [49] found adrenomedullary hyperplasia in sporadic patients. Other authors found bilaterality in sporadic PCCs (Deftos in 10% of sporadic PCC, the present authors in 1/44 sporadic PCCs). Furthermore, in most adrenalectomy specimens containing PCC, the orthotopic tissues of adrenal medulla and cortex are overgrown by the tumour to such an extent that a reliable assessment of the medullary volume is virtually impossible. Extensive analogies between hereditary and nonhereditary PCC are further shown by an identical expression pattern of opioid and polypeptide hormones as detected by immunocytochemistry; correspondingly, DNA cytophotometry revealed no differences between these two groups [43]. In our opinion, morphological methods are unsuitable to recognize an individual case of PCC associated with the MEN 2 syndrome. This is, however, of little or no clinical significance, since the malignant potential of hereditary PCC, as shown above, is no higher than that of nonhereditary PCC. In addition, most patients will already be identified as having MEN 2 by a previously diagnosed MTC.

Hyperplasia of the Parathyroid Gland

Khairi et al. [3] were the first to point out, in 1975, that the incidence of parathyroid diseases is much lower in MEN 2B than in MEN 2A. Apart from the finding of 'multiple neuromas' in MEN 2B, this was the reason both syndromes were interpreted as separate entities (at first termed MEN 2 and MEN 3). In contrast to all other organs developing hyperplasia and/or neoplasia in the settings of MEN 1, 2A and 2B, the parathyroid gland can not be unequivocally integrated within the family of neuroendocrine tissues (amine precursor uptake and decarboxylation system) [50]. Therefore, the aetiological interpretation of syndromatically associated parathyroid hyperplasia is still in question; it is not convincing to explain it as a consequence of elevated calcitonin secretion (or of increased catecholamine release), since neither patients with nonhereditary MTC nor MEN 2B (nor nonhereditary PCC) have an increased incidence of hyperparathyroidism [51]. Whether other humoral factors are responsible for this hyperplasia, such as those found for MEN 1 by Brandi et al. [52], needs further investigation.

The incidence of parathyroid hyperplasia in MEN 2A patients ranges between 20 and 100% [29]. This variability is due to the fact that, even in cases of histologically unequivocal hyperplasia, normal or only sporadically elevated parathyroid hormone levels are found, without hypercalcaemia or clinical signs of hyperparathyroidism.

Therefore normal basal levels of parathyroid hormone do not exclude parathyroid hyperplasia [53, 54]. The reported incidence of biochemically documented hyperparathyroidism varies between 18 and 85% [55–57]; in a recent comprehensive study by Saad et al. [4], 7 out of 30 MEN 2A patients (23%) exhibited hypercalcaemia and elevated levels of parathyroid hormone, though only 2 patients had clinical manifestations of parathyroid disease (in both cases nephrolithiasis). Therefore, symptomatic hyperparathyroidism was regarded as a rare event in MEN 2A, which is consistent with other studies [29].

Discrepancies in the morphological classification of associated parathyroid changes also contribute to the variability of data on the incidence of parathyroid involvement in MEN 2A. In most individual publications [55, 56], as well as in the monographs of the Armed Forces Institute of Pathology and WHO relevant to the classification of endocrine neoplasias [58, 59], the parathyroid findings observed in MEN 2A are classified as chief cell hyperplasia of usually more than one gland. Several other authors have, however, described parathyroid adenomas occurring simultaneously in different glands or in combination with chief cell hyperplasia [4, 53, 57, 60]. These discrepancies are probably due to a lack of definite histological criteria for a clear discrimination of hyperplastic versus adenomatous-neoplastic parathyroid proliferations [50, 58]. Such a sequence of events has been described for C-cells and adrenomedullary cells and is thought to be responsible for the development of hereditary MTC and hereditary PCC. According to Deftos [2], a similar sequence might occur also in the parathyroid.

In contrast to MEN 2A, most MEN 2B patients will present with neither clinical, biochemical nor histological evidence of parathyroid disease [4]. In a detailed study of 34 parathyroid specimens from 24 patients with MEN 2B, Carney et al. [61] could show normal findings in patients up to the age of 17 years, while in older patients only the typical age-related involution of parathyroid tissue was missing, thus resulting in the histological aspect of mild chief cell hyperplasia. In none of the cases, however, was this phenomenon associated with clinical or laboratory findings of hyperparathyroidism.

a

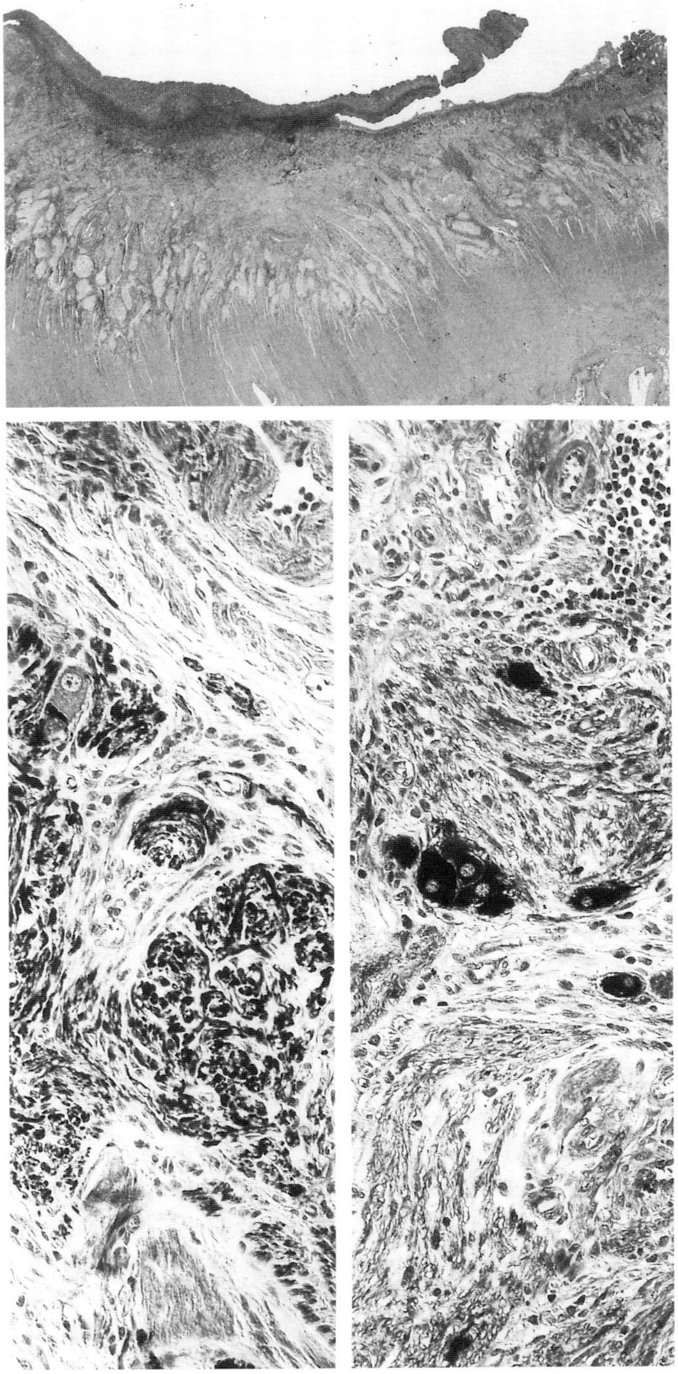

b c

Fig. 4. Ganglioneuromatosis of the small intestine. Low power magnification showing mucosal ulcer and neuroma-like proliferations originating from the submucosal plexus; H&E, ×7.5 (**a**). Higher magnifications demonstrating aggregates of S100-immunoreactive Schwann cells (**b**) and scattered NSE-positive ganglion cells (each ×200) (**c**) (from [68]).

Mucosal Ganglioneuromatosis

Mucosal 'neuromas' associated syndromatically with MTC and adrenal PCC were first described in 1966 by Williams and Pollock [62]. Although these authors correctly recognized the mucosal changes as non-neurofibromatous, they falsely assumed an association with von Recklinghausen's neurofibromatosis. In 1968, Gorlin et al. [63] defined the complete syndrome of MEN 2B as it is accepted today, including the ocular findings and the marfanoid appearance, in a synopsis of 17 cases – including the 11 patients presented two years earlier by Williams and Pollock [62].

Tumour-like neural proliferations in MEN 2B patients are a diagnostic finding, particularly in the centrofacial parts of the oral mucosa (i.e. lips, tongue, buccal regions, gingiva, pharynx and palate) [3]. The diagnostic significance of these findings is emphasized by the observations of Carney and Hayles [64], who found that 7 out of 17 MEN 2B patients already showed mucosal changes at birth and another 6 patients developed them before the age of 6 years, and, in 14 out of 17 patients, oral lesions preceded the endocrine tumours. The oral manifestations are followed by ocular (cornea, conjunctiva and eyelid) lesions, and gastrointestinal lesions with the histological appearance of ganglioneuromatosis already described by Williams and Pollock [62]. According to Carney and Hayles [64] and d'Amore et al. [65], in contrast to Khairi et al. [3], intestinal lesions can also be regarded as a diagnostic finding in MEN 2B. The mucosae of nose and larynx [3], bronchi and urinary bladder [66] are reported as comparatively rare extragastrointestinal localizations of ganglioneuromatosis.

Histologically, the oral and ocular mucosal changes have been diversely diagnosed by different authors as neurofibromas, plexiform neurofibromas, myelinated neuromas and neuromas. According to Carney et al. [67], however, all these terms are inappropriate, since the extragastrointestinal, as well as the gastrointestinal, lesions do not consist of neoplastic, but of hamartomatous proliferations of nerve fibres, Schwann cells and occasionally also ganglion cells (fig. 4). Thus, quantitative, but no qualitative, discrepancies exist between the extragastrointestinal and gastrointestinal manifestations of MEN 2B. The term 'diffuse ganglioneuromatosis' should, therefore, also be used to designate the oral and ocular lesions in MEN 2B.

Acknowledgement

This work was supported by the Deutsche Forschungsgemeinschaft and the Hamburger Krebsgesellschaft.

References

1 Heitz PU Steiner H: Pluriglanduläre endokrine Regulationsstörungen; in Doerr W, Seifert G (eds): Pathologie der Endokrinen Organe (Spezielle pathologische Anatomie). Berlin, Springer, 1981, 14 ii, pp 1137–1203.
2 Deftos LJ: Medullary Thyroid Carcinoma. Basel, Karger, 1983.
3 Khairi MRA, Dexter RN, Burzynski NJ, et al: Mucosal neuroma, pheochromocytoma and medullary thyroid carcinoma: Multiple endocrine neoplasia type 3. Medicine 1975;54:89–112.
4 Saad MF, Ordonez NG, Rashid RK, et al: Medullary carcinoma of the thyroid. A study of the clinical features and prognostic factors in 161 patients. Medicine 1984;63:319–342.
5 Schröder S, Böcker W, Baisch H, et al: Prognostic factors in medullary thyroid carcinomas: Survival in relation to age, sex, stage, histology, immunocytochemistry and DNA content. Cancer 1988;62:806–816.
6 Bergholm U, Adami HO, Auer G, et al: Histopathologic characteristics and nuclear DNA content as prognostic factors in medullary thyroid carcinoma. A nationwide study in Sweden. Cancer 1989;64:135–142.
7 Bigner SH, Mendelsohn G, Wells SA, et al: Medullary carcinoma of the thyroid in the multiple endocrine neoplasia IIA syndrome. Am J Surg Pathol 1981;5:459–472.
8 Hedinger C: Histological Typing of Thyroid Tumours. International Histological Classification of Tumours. No. 11. 2nd ed. Berlin, Springer, 1988.
9 Wolfe HJ, Lelvin KEW, Cervi-Skinner SJ, et al: C-cell hyperplasia preceding medullary thyroid carcinoma. N Engl J Med 1973;289:437–441.
10 DeLellis RA, Nunnemacher G, Wolfe HJ: C-cell hyperplasia. An ultrastructural analysis. Lab Invest 1977;36:237–248.
11 Schröder S, Klöppel G: Carcinoembryonic antigen and nonspecific cross-reacting antigens in thyroid cancer. An immunocytochemical study using polyclonal and monoclonal antibodies. Am J Surg Pathol 1987;11:100–108.
12 Baylin SB, Mendelsohn G, Weisburger WR, et al: Levels of histaminase and L-dopa decarboxylase activity in the transition from C-cell hyperplasia to familial medullary thyroid carcinoma. Cancer 1979;44:1315–1321.
13 Wolfe HJ, DeLellis RA, Jackson CE, et al: Immunocytochemical distinction of hereditary from sporadic medullary thyroid carcinoma. Lab Invest 1980;42:161–162.
14 Ulbright TM, Kraus FT, O'Neal LW: C-cell hyperplasia developing in residual thyroid following resection of sporadic medullary carcinoma. Cancer 1981;48:2076–2079.
15 Uribe M, Fenoglio-Preiser CM, Grimes M, et al: Medullary carcinoma of the thyroid gland: Clinical, pathological and immunohistochemical features with review of the literature. Am J Surg Pathol 1985;9:577–594.
16 Rosenberg-Bourgin M, Gardet P, de Sahb R, et al: Comparison of sporadic and hereditary forms of medullary thyroid carcinoma. Henry Ford Hosp Med J 1989;37:141–143.
17 Albores-Saavedra J, Monforte H, Nadji M, et al: C-cell hyperplasia in thyroid tissue adjacent to follicular cell tumors. Hum Pathol 1988;19:795–799.
18 Libbey NP, Nowakowski KJ, Tucci JR: C-cell hyperplasia of the thyroid in a patient with goitrous hypothyroidism and Hashimoto's thyroiditis. Am J Surg Pathol 1989;13:71–77.
19 Biddinger PW, Brennan MF, Rosen PP: Symptomatic C-cell hyperplasia associated with chronic lymphocytic thyroiditis. Am J Surg Pathol 1991;15:599–604.
20 Gibson WGH, Peng T, Croker BP: Age-associated C-cell hyperplasia in the human thyroid. Am J Pathol 1982;106:388–393.
21 Lips CJM, Leo JR, Berends MJH: Thyroid C-cell hyperplasia and micronodules in close relatives of MEN-2A patients: Pitfalls in early diagnosis and reevaluation of criteria for surgery. Henry Ford Hosp Med J 1987;35:133–138.

22 Raue F: Rundschreiben 9/90 der Deutschen Studiengruppe Medulläres Schilddrüsencarcinom 1990.
23 Carney JA, Roth SI, Heath H, et al: The parathyroid glands in multiple endocrine neoplasia, type 2b. Cancer 1979;44:2173–2183.
24 Norton JA, Froome LC, Farrell RE, et al: Multiple endocrine neoplasia type IIb. The most aggressive form of medullary thyroid carcinoma. Surg Clin N Am 1979;59:109–118.
25 Jackson CE, Talpos GB, Kambouris A, et al: The clinical course after definitive operation for medullary thyroid carcinoma. Surgery 1983;94:995–1001.
26 Samaan NA, Schultz PN, Hickey RC: Medullary thyroid carcinoma: Prognosis of familial versus nonfamilial disease and the role of radiotherapy. Horm Metab Res 1989;Suppl 21:21–25.
27 Kakudo K, Carney JA, Sizemore GW: Medullary carcinoma of the thyroid. Biological behaviour of the sporadic and familial neoplasms. Cancer 1985;55:2818–2821.
28 Thompson NW: Commentary following Jackson CE, Talpos GB, Block MA, Norum RA, Lloyd RV, Tashjian AH: Clinical value of tumor doubling estimations in multiple endocrine neoplasia type II. Surgery 1984;96: 981–987.
29 Grün R, Eberle F: Multiple endocrine neoplasia, type II (MEN II). Ergebn Inn Med Kinderheilkd 1981;46:151–201.
30 Carney JA, Sizemore GW, Sheps SG: Adrenal medullary disease in multiple endocrine neoplasia, type 2. Pheochromocytoma and its precursors. Am J Clin Pathol 1976;66:279–290.
31 DeLellis RA, Wolfe HJ, Gagel RF, et al: Adrenal medullary hyperplasia. A morphometric analysis in patients with familial medullary thyroid carcinoma. Am J Pathol 1976;83: 177–196.
32 Symington T: Functional Pathology of the Human Adrenal Gland. Baltimore, Williams and Wilkins, 1969, pp 13–14.
33 Webb TA, Sheps SG, Carney JA: Differences between sporadic pheochromocytoma and pheochromocytoma in multiple endocrine neoplasia, type 2. Am J Surg Pathol 1980;4: 121–126.
34 Lips CJM, van der Sluys Veer J, Struyvenberg A, et al: Bilateral occurrence of pheochromocytoma in patients with the multiple endocrine neoplasia syndrome, type 2A (Sipple's syndrome). Am J Med 1981;70:1051–1060.
35 Rosai J: Adrenal gland and other paragangliomas; in Rosai J (ed): Ackerman's Surgical Pathology. 7th ed. St Louis, Mosby, 1989, vol 1, pp 789–818.
36 van Heerden JA, Shep SH, Hamberger B, et al: Pheochromocytoma: Current status and changing trends. Surgery 1982;91:367–373.
37 Scott HW, Halter SA: Oncologic aspects of pheochromocytoma: The importance of follow-up. Surgery 1984;96:1061–1066.
38 Stenström G, Ernest I, Tisell LE: Long-term results in 64 patients operated upon for pheochromocytoma. Acta Med Scand 1988;223: 345–352.
39 Westfried M, Mandel D, Alderete MN, et al: Sipple's syndrome with a malignant pheochromocytoma presenting as a pericardial effusion. Cardiology 1978;63:305–311.
40 Carney JA, Go VLW, Sizemore GW, et al: Alimentary tract ganglioneuromatosis. A major component of the syndrome of multiple endocrine neoplasia, type 2b. N Engl J Med 1976;295:1287–1291.
41 Wilson RA, Ibanez ML: A comparative study of 14 cases of familial and nonfamilial pheochromocytomas. Hum Pathol 1978;9:181–188.
42 Samaan NA, Hickey RC, Shutts PE: Diagnosis, localization, and management of pheochromocytoma. Pitfalls and follow-up in 41 patients. Cancer 1988;62:2451–2460.
43 Padberg B, Achilles E, Garbe E, et al: Histologie, Immuncytochemie und DNA-cytophotometrie des adrenalen Phäochromocytoms (PCC) – eine morphologisch-klinische Untersuchung an 64 Tumoren. Verh Dtsch Ges Pathol 1990;74:289–294.
44 Graeff J de, Muller H, Moolenaar AJ: Pheochromocytoma. A report of seven cases. Acta Med Scand 1959;164:419–430.
45 Marks AD, Channick BJ: Extra-adrenal pheochromocytoma and medullary thyroid carcinoma with pheochromocytoma. Arch Int Med 1974;134:1106–1109.
46 Lips CJM, Minder WH, Leo JR, et al: Evidence of multicentric origin of the multiple endocrine neoplasia syndrome type 2A (Sipple's syndrome) in a large family in the Netherlands. Diagnostic and therapeutic implications. Am J Med 1978;64:569–578.
47 Lloyd RV, Blaivas M, Wilson BS: Distribution of chromogranin and S100 protein in normal and abnormal adrenal medullary tissues. Arch Pathol Lab Med 1985;109:633–635.
48 Achilles E, Padberg BC, Holl K, et al: Immunocytochemistry of paragangliomas – value of S100 and GFAP staining in diagnosis and prognosis. Histopathology 1991;18:453–458.
49 Dralle H, Schröder S, Gratz KF, et al: Sporadic unilateral adrenomedullary hyperplasia with hypertension cured by adrenalectomy. World J Surg 1990;14:308–316.
50 Altenähr E: Nebenschilddrüsen; in Doerr W, Seifert G (eds): Pathologie der Endokrinen Organe (Spezielle pathologische Anatomie). Berlin, Springer, 1981, 14 i, pp 417–521.
51 Raue F, Gagel RF: Multiple 'endokrine' Neoplasie; in Hesch RD (ed): Endokrinologie. München, Urban and Schwarzenberg, 1989, pp 1109–1116.
52 Brandi ML, Aurbach GD, Fitzpatrick LA, et al: Parathyroid mitogenic activity in plasma from patients with familial multiple endocrine neoplasia type 1. N Engl J Med 1986;314: 1287–1293.
53 Block MA, Jackson CE, Tashjian AH: Management of parathyroid glands in surgery for medullary thyroid carcinoma. Arch Surg 1975; 110:617–624.
54 Heath H, Sizemore GW, Carney JA: Preoperative diagnosis of occult parathyroid hyperplasia by calcium infusion in patients with multiple endocrine neoplasia, type 2a. J Clin Endocrinol Metab 1976;43:428–435.
55 Keiser HR, Beaven MA, Doppman S, et al: Sipple's syndrome: Medullary thyroid carcinoma, pheochromocytoma, and parathyroid disease. Studies in a large family. Ann Intern Med 1973;78:561–579.
56 Melvin KEW, Tasjian AH, Miller HH: Studies in a familial (medullary) thyroid carcinoma. Rec Prog Horm Res 1972;28:399–470.
57 Steiner AL, Goodman AD, Powers SR: Study of a kindred with pheochromocytoma, medullary thyroid carcinoma, hyperparathyroidism, and Cushing's disease: MEN, type II. Medicine 1968;47:371–409.
58 Castleman B, Roth SI: Tumors of the Parathyroid Glands. Atlas of Tumor Pathology. 2nd series, Fasc 14. Washington DC, Armed Forces Institute of Pathology, 1978.
59 Williams ED, Siebenmann RE, Sobin LH: Histological Typing of Endocrine Tumours. International Histological Classification of Tumours. No 23. Geneva, World Health Organization, 1980.
60 Sarosi G, Doe RP: Familial occurrence of parathyroid adenomas, pheochromocytoma, and medullary carcinoma of the thyroid with amyloid stroma (Sipple's syndrome). Arch Intern Med 1968;68:1305–1309.
61 Carney JA, Roth SI, Heath H, et al: The parathyroid glands in multiple endocrine neoplasia type 2b. Am J Pathol 1980;99:387–398.
62 Williams ED, Pollock DJ: Multiple mucosal neuromata with endocrine tumours. A syndrome allied to von Recklinghausen's disease. J Pathol Bacteriol 1966;91:71–80.
63 Gorlin RJ, Sedano HO, Vickers RA, et al: Multiple mucosal neuromas, pheochromocytomas, and medullary carcinoma of the thyroid – a syndrome. Cancer 1968;22:293–299.
64 Carney JA, Hayles AB: Alimentary tract manifestations of multiple endocrine neoplasia, type 2b. Mayo Clin Proc 1977;52:543–548.
65 d'Amore ES, Manivel JC, Pettinato G, et al: Intestinal ganglioneuromatosis: Mucosal and transmural types. Hum Pathol 1991;22: 276–286.
66 Schimke RN, Hartmann WH, Prout TE, et al: Syndrome of bilateral pheochromocytoma, medullary thyroid carcinoma, and multiple neuromas. N Engl J Med 1968;279:1–7.
67 Carney JA, Sizemore GW, Lovestedt SA: Mucosal ganglioneuromatosis, medullary thyroid carcinoma, and pheochromocytoma: Multiple endocrine neoplasia, type 2b. Oral Surg 1976;41:739–752.
68 Schröder S, Padberg BC: Pathologie der multiplen endokrinen Neoplasien 2A and 2B – eine aktuelle Bestandsaufnahme. Pathologe 1991; 12:131–137.

Horm Res 1992;38(suppl 2):31–35

F. Raue
A. Zink

Department of Internal Medicine I –
Endocrinology and Metabolism,
University of Heidelberg, Germany

Clinical Features of Multiple Endocrine Neoplasia Type 1 and Type 2

Key Words
Wermer's syndrome
Sipple's syndrome
MEN 1
MEN 2a
MEN 2b
Parathyroid tumour
Pancreatic islet cell tumour
Pituitary tumour
Medullary thyroid carcinoma
Phaeochromocytoma
Screening

Abstract

The term 'Multiple Endocrine Neoplasia' (MEN) denotes a genetically determined syndrome characterized by the independent appearance of benign or malignant changes of several endocrine organs as well as occasional changes of neural, muscular and connective tissue. Three different forms have been identified: MEN 1 (Wermer's syndrome) includes parathyroid hyperplasia in combination with pancreatic islet cell and pituitary tumours; MEN 2a (Sipple's syndrome) includes medullary thyroid carcinoma in association with phaeochromocytoma and parathyroid hyperplasia; MEN 2b includes medullary thyroid carcinoma, phaeochromocytoma and mucosal neuromas. MEN syndrome is transmitted as an autosomal dominant trait with a high degree of penetrance. The changes in the individual glands appear to be causally and temporally independent of each other. A spectrum of pathological changes exist in the affected glands which range from hyperplasia to adenoma to carcinoma. The pathological process is almost always multicentric, often resulting in bilateral disease of organs. The appearance of an endocrine tumour known to be associated with MEN should alert the physician to the possibility of a MEN syndrome. When the possibility of such a syndrome exists, screening and long-term observation should be initiated to diagnose a carcinoma in its earliest stage, or before the development of clinical manifestations of hormone excess.

Introduction

'Multiple Endocrine Neoplasia' (MEN) is a genetically determined syndrome characterized by the independent appearance of benign or malignant changes of two or more endocrine glands as well as occasional changes of neuronal, muscular and connective tissue. Despite widely varying manifestations, two major forms of MEN have been identified, type 1 and type 2. MEN 1 (also called Wermer's syndrome) is characterized by the combined occurrence of tumours in the parathyroid glands, pancreatic islet cells and the pituitary. MEN 2 (also called Sipple's syndrome) has three variants, MEN 2a, MEN 2b and medullary thyroid carcinoma (MTC)-only [1, 2]. In MEN 2a, the most common variant, the development of MTC is associated with phaeochromocytoma and hyperplasia of the parathyroid glands. However, in MEN 2b parathyroid involvement is absent and the occurrence of MTC and phaeochromocy-

F. Raue
Department of Internal Medicine I
Endocrinology and Metabolism
University of Heidelberg, Bergheimerstrasse 58
D-W-6900 Heidelberg (Germany)

0301–0163/92/0388–0031
$ 2.75/0

toma is associated with a marfanoid habitus and mucosal neuromas. In the third variant, MTC is the only manifestation of the syndrome [3, 4].

The MEN syndrome is transmitted as an autosomal dominant trait with a high degree of penetrance, though not every family member affected will develop all of the polyglandular neoplasia manifestations for the particular syndrome [1]. The changes in the individual glands appear temporally independent of each other. A spectrum of pathological changes exists in the affected glands, which range from hyperplasia to adenoma to carcinoma. The carcinomatous state is almost always multicentric, often resulting in bilateral disease. The appearance of an endocrine tumour known to be associated with MEN should alert the physician to the possibility of an MEN syndrome, and screening should be initiated to diagnose other manifestations of MEN.

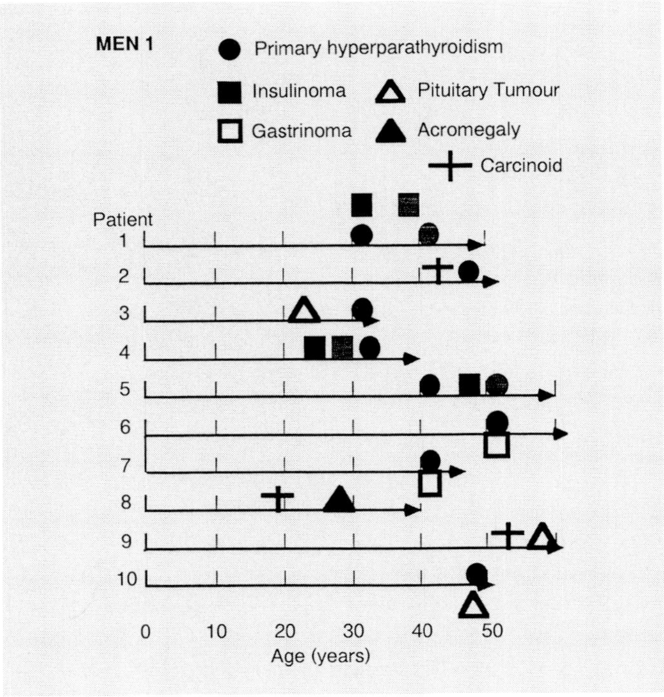

Fig. 1. Clinical presentation of 10 patients with MEN 1.

Clinical Presentation of MEN 1

The clinical presentation of patients with MEN 1 depends on the site of organ involvement and hormone secretion. This disorder affects virtually all age groups with an average range of 20–60 years. Expression of MEN 1 is uncommon before the age of 10, typically beginning between 20 and 40 years; 80% of patients have presented by the fifth decade (fig. 1). Primary hyperparathyroidism is the most common and often also the first lesion to become clinically detected. Hyperfunction of the parathyroids develops in 95% of patients with MEN 1, 30–80% of patients develop pancreatic tumours and 15–90% get pituitary tumours. These are the major components of MEN 1; adrenal cortical tumours, carcinoid and lipomatous tumours have occasionally been described [1].

Parathyroid Tumour

Primary hyperparathyroidism is an important feature of MEN 1 and occurs in more than 95% of all MEN 1 patients. Conversely, only 3% of all cases of primary hyperparathyroidism are associated with the framework of MEN 1 or MEN 2. The clinical presentation of primary hyperparathyroidism in MEN 1 is not different from that associated with the independent form. A family history suggestive of hypercalcaemia or kidney stones should lead to an appropriate screening of the patient and family. The possibility of familial disease should also be considered when chief cell hyperplasia, multiple parathyroid adenomas, or a postoperative persistence or recurrence of hypercalcaemia suggest a multifocal process. Asymptomatic hypercalcaemia is most common, with only 20–30% of patients presenting with definite hypercalcaemic signs or symptoms. Diagnosis is confirmed by finding hypercalcaemia associated with elevated intact parathyroid hormone (PTH) in the circulation. Total parathyroidectomy with autotransplantation of parathyroid tissue in the forearm is recommended. Because of the high rate of recurrence of hyperparathyroidism (41% by 10 years), regular postoperative, long-term measurements of serum calcium are necessary.

Pancreatic Islet Cell Tumour

Gastrinoma (Zollinger-Ellison syndrome, ZES) represents over 50% of all pancreatic islet cell tumours in MEN 1 and are the major cause of morbidity and mortality of MEN 1 patients. However, about 50% of all patients with ZES are likely to have MEN 1. The malignancy rate of gastrinoma associated with MEN 1 is 50% and similar to the independent form of the disease. Clinically, patients with ZES present with complications of peptic ulcer disease, such as epigastric pain, gastrointestinal bleeding, perforation and diarrhoea. Diagnosis is made by demonstration of a raised fasting serum gastrin concentration in association with an increased basal gastric acid secretion.

Medical treatment with a proton pump inhibitor, such as omeprazole, is the therapy of choice for pharmacological control of gastric acid hypersecretion. If a solitary tumour is identified by imaging methods, it is reasonable to attempt surgical removal. Efforts to cure gastrinoma in MEN 1 by surgery have largely been unsuccessful because of multiple islet tumours, extrapancreatic primary sites (e.g. the duodenal submucosa) or early metastasis. A total gastrectomy is indicated when pharmacological forms of therapy are inadequate to control the ulcer diathesis. Primary hyperparathyroidism can exacerbate acid-peptic disease in ZES, so in patients with gastrinoma and primary hyperparathyroidism, parathyroidectomy is highly recommended. One third of the islet cell tumours are insulinomas which may occur in association with gastrinomas. Symptoms are typical of neuroglycopenia which develop after an overnight fast and improve after glucose intake. Biochemical investigation reveals raised plasma insulin concentration in association with hypoglycaemia. If surgical treatment, which ranges from enucleation of a single tumour to partial pancreatectomy, is not successful, medical treatment with diazoxide may be required. Glucagenoma and vipoma are rare pancreatic tumours in MEN 1, their clinical symptoms are related to their hormone secretions. PPomas secrete pancreatic polypeptide but no clinical syndrome is associated with the excessive pancreatic polypeptide secretion.

Pituitary Tumours

The incidence of pituitary tumours in MEN 1 patients varies widely (from 15 to 90%) in different series. The most common type is prolactinoma, followed by growth hormone secreting tumour and a hormone-inactive pituitary tumour. ACTH-producing tumours seldom occur. Prolactinoma may cause amenorrhoea, infertility and galactorrhoea. Medical treatment with bromocriptine has been effective in decreasing tumour size, decreasing serum prolactin levels and restoring gonadal function. Growth hormone secreting tumours cause acromegaly. Microsurgical tumour extirpation is the treatment of choice. Pituitary insufficiency should be treated with appropriate hormone replacement.

Screening for MEN 1

The appearance of an endocrine tumour known to be associated with MEN should alert physicians to the possibility of an MEN syndrome. When this possibility exists, screening and long-term observation of the patient and their relatives should be initiated to allow early diagnosis of a life threatening tumour or carcinoma before clinical manifestations or hormone excess develop. Therefore, the members of MEN 1 families must undergo repeated screening examinations every one or two years. All individuals over 10 years of age should have a physical examination and a fasting blood sample taken for measurement of serum calcium, PTH (for detection of parathyroid tumours), gastrin, insulin and blood glucose (for detection of pancreatic tumours), and prolactin and growth hormone (for pituitary tumours) (table 1) [5]. If a pathological basal value is revealed in any of these tests, standard meal test and/or a pituitary test is performed. Using this screening procedure Öberg and colleagues [5] were able to reduce the age of diagnosis by almost two decades to an average of 18 years. The early detection and surgical intervention will probably result in an impact on morbidity and perhaps mortality of affected members of MEN 1 families. Localization of the MEN 1 gene on chromosome 11 and established genetic markers will also facilitate the indication of gene carriers. Those with a low probability of being gene carriers can probably be excluded from screening [6].

Table 1. Parameters for screening in MEN 1

Parameter	Tumour to be detected
S-calcium intact PTH	Parathyroid tumour
Gastrin	Gastrinoma
Insulin, blood glucose	Insulinoma
Prolactin	Prolactinoma
Growth hormone	Acromegaly

Clinical Presentation of MEN 2a

The most common manifestation in MEN 2 is the medullary thyroid carcinoma (MTC) which derives from calcitonin-producing parafollicular C-cells. 75% of MTC occurs in a sporadic (nonhereditary) form, and 25% in one of three familial (hereditary) forms, distinguished by the other tissues involved and the aggressiveness of the disease [7]. The most common familial form is MEN 2a, the combination of MTC with unilateral or bilateral phaeochromocytoma and multiple parathyroid adenomas. The MTC-only presentation is also common, here MTC is the sole manifestation and may represent an incomplete expression of the MEN 2a gene. In MEN 2b, MTC and phaeochromocytoma may be combined with a marfanoid habitus and multiple neuromas (fig.2). In these families the condition is inherited as an autosomal dominant trait with incomplete penetrance [8]. Thus, many patients may have inherited the disease from a parent who, though elder, does not have clinical symptoms. Of those who present clinically at diagnosis (index cases) nearly half die of the disease and many more suffer significant morbidity.

Medullary Thyroid Carcinoma

The clinical presentation of familial MTC (index cases) does not differ from nonhereditary MTC. These clinical signs include the development of a cold thyroid nodule detected by thyroid scan or the appearance of a clinical syndrome caused by hypersecretion of one or more hormones by the tumour, for example, ACTH hypersecretion causes Cushing's syndrome. The mean age of onset of clinical symptoms is about 40 years.

Diffuse C-cell hyperplasia, the premalignant lesion and the hallmark of the disease in MEN 2, may persist for years before the development of a multicentric carcinoma. It is now possible to detect C-cell hyperplasia or microcarcinoma consistently by prospective screening of potentially affected family members at an early stage, before metastatic disease develops. Measurement of serum calcitonin after administration of pentagastrin, which stimulates calcitonin release, is the clue for the early diagnosis of MTC. In patients detected by this method, the clinical presentation is silent [9].

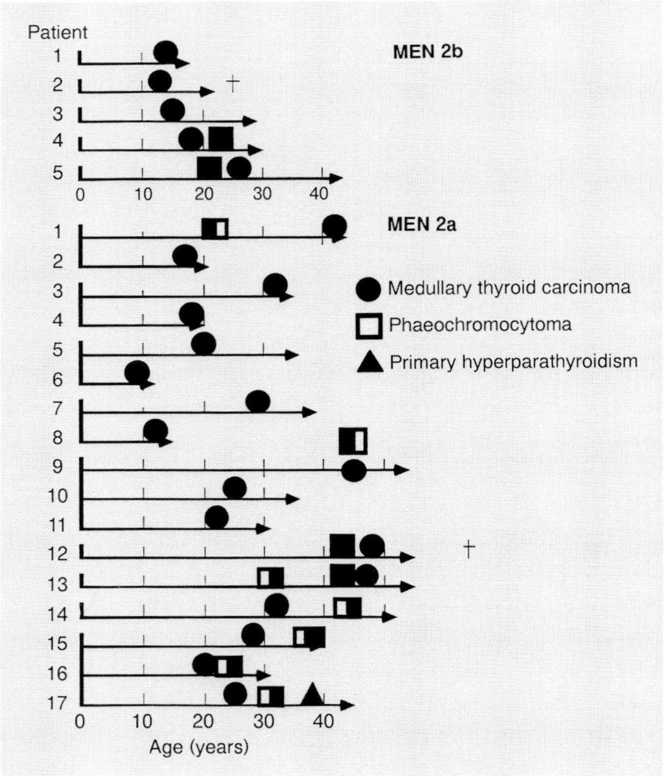

Fig. 2. Clinical presentation of 23 patients with MEN 2.

Phaeochromocytoma

Of individuals affected with MEN 2a, 50% will develop unilateral or bilateral phaeochromocytoma. In most cases, diagnosis of adrenal medullary disease follows the identification of MTC. Conversely, only 5% of all phaeochromocytomas appear to be familial, and of these, 20% occur in MEN 2. Typically, phaeochromocytomas are bilateral but never extra-adrenal. The malignancy rate is less than 10% of that of sporadic phaeochromocytoma. The clinical manifestations of phaeochromocytoma occurring as part of MEN 2 are usually subtle, more than 50% of patients with phaeochromocytoma are asymptomatic and normotensive.

The biochemical diagnosis of phaeochromocytoma can be made by serum and/or by urine catecholamine determination. In all patients in whom MTC is diagnosed, studies of catecholamine excess should be performed to exclude adrenal medullary disease, particularly before any operation is planned. Conversely, in patients with bilateral and/or familial phaeochromocytoma a pentagastrin stimulation test is recommended to exclude MTC.

Phaeochromocytoma can be localized by sonography, computed tomography or magnetic resonance imaging. ^{131}I-metaiodo benzyl-guanidine (MIBG) scintigraphy provides a noninvasive specific technique for localization of catecholamine-producing tumour. The diagnosis of phaeochromocytoma can be made by MIBG scintigraphy even before the appearance of increased urinary excretion of catecholamines.

Parathyroid Tumour

The third and least common component of the MEN 2 syndrome is primary hyperparathyroidism. This manifestation is observed in 10–20% of patients with the fully developed syndrome. The majority of patients have no clinical or biochemical evidence of disease, even though hyperplasia of removed parathyroid glandular tissue may be found at thyroidectomy for MTC. Annual screening of serum calcium and for elevated intact PTH seems to be sufficient for early diagnosis.

Clinical Presentation of MEN 2b

The distinctive feature of MEN 2b syndrome is the marfanoid habitus, with long thin extremities and the characteristic facies with thickened lips. The cause of these bumpy lips are mucosal neuromas located in a centrofacial distribution on the tongue and lips. They are also found on the eyelids and the conjunctiva [10]. The neuromas may be present throughout the gastrointestinal tract in combination with disordered autonomic ganglia in the wall of the gut. This may lead to gastrointestinal symptoms, including intestinal obstruction. The characteristic phenotypic appearance of the patients, even in infancy, should alert the physicians to the diagnosis of MEN 2b. The performance of a pentagastrin test for calcitonin release will generally confirm the diagnosis of MTC.

The prognosis in the MEN 2b syndrome is generally poor as a result of an aggressive MTC, that develops earlier in life than in patients with MEN 2a. Survival times are similar to the nonhereditary MTC (5 years: 78%; 10 years: 59%), while MEN 2a and only-MTC have a much better prognosis with 5-year and 10-year survival rates of 86 and 72%, respectively. This can be improved by regular screening of patients of risk; early diagnosis allows thyroidectomy and/or adrenalectomy which is likely to be curative.

Screening for MEN 2

Family screening has to be considered for every new patient with MTC, and for apparently sporadic cases. Calcitonin determination after stimulation with pentagastrin is the 'gold standard' for family screening to detect premalignant lesions (C-cell hyperplasia) (table 2). To identify these patients with early forms of MTC, testing of close blood relatives should start at the age of 3–4 years and continue annually until the age of 35 or until a positive test result could be confirmed [11]. The likelihood of conversion to positive after 35 years of age is less than 5%, so it seems reasonable to reduce the frequency of testing after that age. Not all patients with genetically determined disease will present with MTC, indicating incomplete penetrance, but virtually all have a positive test by the age of 35 years. Setting up a systematic annual screening programme in MEN 2 families permits morbidity and mortality to be reduced by early thyroidectomy which is likely to be curative at that stage. Of patients presenting with clinical signs, 87% already have metastases at diagnosis and can not be cured. Postoperative calcitonin levels are elevated in 75% of cases, while patients detected by follow-up screening had no metastasis and could all be cured [9]. Systematic screening of this type has reduced the age of diagnosis of familial MTC to about 15 years. Biochemical screening combined with genetic screening by DNA markers will improve the sensitivity and accuracy of the overall screening process [12].

Table 2. Parameters for screening in MEN 2

Parameter	Tumour to be detected
Calcitonin after pentagastrin stimulation	Medullary thyroid carcinoma
Catecholamines (serum, urine)	Phaeochromocytoma
S-calcium, intact PTH	Parathyroid tumour

References

1 Thakker RV, Ponder BAJ: Multiple endocrine neoplasia. Baillière's Clinical Endocr Metab 1988;2:1031–1067.
2 Marx SJ: Familial multiple endocrine neoplasia type 1. TEM 1989;1:76–82.
3 Gagel RF, Tashjian AH, Cummings T, et al: The clinical outcome of prospective screening for multiple endocrine neoplasia type 2a, and 18-year experience. N Engl J Med 1988;318: 478–484.
4 Raue F, Gagel RF: Multiple endocrine Neoplasie; in Hesch RD (ed): Endokrinologie II, Innere Medizin der Gegenwart. München, Urban und Schwarzenberg Verlag, 1989, pp 1073–1079.
5 Skogseid B, Eriksson B, Lundquist G, et al: Multiple endocrine neoplasia type 1: A 10-year prospective screening study in four kindreds. J Clin Endocr Metab 1991;73:281–287.
6 Larsson K, Skogseid B, Öberg K, et al: Multiple endocrine neoplasia type 1 gene maps to chromosome 11 and is lost in insulinoma. Nature 1988;332:85–87.
7 Raue F, Späth-Röger M, Winter J, et al: Register für das medulläre Schilddrüsencarcinom in der Bundesrepublik Deutschland. Med Klinik 1990;3:113–116.
8 Grün R, Eberle F: Multiple endocrine neoplasia type II (MEN II). Ergeb Inn Med Kinderheilk 1981;46:151–201.
9 Vasen HFA, Nieuwenhuyzen-Krusemann AC, Berkel H, et al: Multiple endocrine neoplasia syndrome type 2: The value of screening and central registration, a study of 15 kindreds in The Netherlands. Am J Med 1987;83:847–852.
10 Frank K, Raue F, Gottswinter J, et al: Importance of early diagnosis and follow-up in multiple endocrine neoplasia (MEN IIB). Europ J Pediat 1984;143:112–116.
11 Ponder BA, Ponder MA, Coffey R, et al: Risk estimation and screening in families of patients with medullary thyroid carcinoma. Lancet 1988;i:397–401.
12 Mathew CG, Chin KS, Easton DF, et al: A linked genetic marker for multiple endocrine neoplasia type 2A on chromosome 10. Nature 1987;328:527–528.

Horm Res 1992;38(suppl 2):36

P. Saenger

Introduction

The second workshop of this meeting reviews the anabolic and metabolic effects of growth hormone (GH) action. Catabolic states characterizing acute or chronic illness, postoperative states and burns, are often difficult to treat with nutritional support therapy alone. Ever since the early work of Wilmore's group addressing the efficacy of human growth and high calorific feeding in reversing the catabolic states after thermal injury, there has been increasing interest from internists, surgeons, and paediatricians in reversing the catabolic states with GH.

Dr David Clemmons and his co-workers at the University of North Carolina School of Medicine, Chapel Hill, have been major contributors in this field. While many patients respond to daily GH, albeit at doses 5–10 times higher than those used for the treatment of GH deficiency, others prove to be resistant to the nitrogen sparing effects of GH. In a rational extension, therefore, recent research focuses on the efficacy of IGF-I in overcoming resistance to the anabolic effects of GH. Since GH and IGF-I have diametrically opposed effects on carbohydrate tolerance (GH leading to insulin resistance while IGF-I may cause hypoglycaemia), a combination of both drugs may turn out to be the most promising avenue for future research.

In the second presentation Dr Gertner, Cornell University Medical College, New York, presents data investigating the GH-fat cycle. Beyond the well-known acute lipolytic effect of GH, the free fatty acid concentration may participate in a negative feedback loop modulating GH release. Indeed, obese children secrete much less GH than age-matched controls. Higher IGF-I levels measured in obese children – who are in most instances also taller than average – may contribute to the inhibitory effect of obesity on GH release. A direct extension of these observations is the experimental use of GH in treating obesity. Further studies probing the GH-fat cycle will hopefully tie together the dual effects of GH in this context – longitudinal growth and weight control.

Dr Morey Haymond, University of Florida, Jacksonville, explores the effects of GH in the catabolic states caused by glucocorticoids. As high-dose glucocorticoids frequently represent the only therapeutic modalities in many chronic diseases, decrease or reversal of attendant nitrogen losses would be desirable. Using sophisticated techniques, such as isotope dilution techniques employing labelled leucine, Dr Haymond studied the action of cortisol and GH on whole body protein metabolism.

It has always been an assumption that GH affects de novo protein synthesis via the generation of IGF-I. With the recent availability of recombinant hIGF-I, the different effects of GH and IGF-I on protein synthesis and proteolysis can now be studied for the first time. To date, Dr Haymond and his colleagues have shown convincingly that GH at high doses can prevent the protein catabolic effects of steroids in humans.

Dr Bill Tamborlane, Yale University, New Haven, applies state-of-the-art techniques to the examination of developmental changes in insulin secretion and action during childhood. The effects of GH on carbohydrate tolerance have to be viewed against the backdrop of physiological decreases in insulin sensitivity occurring during adolescence. Indeed, the augmented insulin responses in normal adolescence are presumably mediated through the well-known increased GH secretory activity in adolescence. It is particularly intriguing that carbohydrate intolerance in adolescence is chiefly an impairment in peripheral and not hepatic glucose uptake. Furthermore, the augmented insulin response in teenagers leads to a greater fall in branched chain amino acids and other essential amino acids. Thus, the hyperinsulinaemia may serve as a beneficial effect by amplifying the anabolic effects of insulin on protein metabolism – teleologically a welcome metabolic change during the pubertal growth spurt. Preliminary data suggest that GH treatment in idiopathic short stature leads to identical changes in glucose, amino acid metabolism and insulin responses as are seen during normal puberty in healthy controls.

In addressing the important issue of the potential adverse effects of GH treatment, these four presentations provide a comprehensive review of the anabolic and metabolic effects of GH and IGF-I.

Horm Res 1992;38(suppl 2):37–40

D.R. Clemmons
L.E. Underwood

Departments of Medicine and Pediatrics,
University of North Carolina,
Chapel Hill, NC, USA

Role of Insulin-Like Growth Factors and Growth Hormone in Reversing Catabolic States

Key Words
Nitrogen balance
Somatomedin-C
Anabolism
Muscle mass

Abstract
The insulin-like growth factors (IGFs) mediate the anabolic effects of growth hormone or protein synthesis in muscle and skeletal tissues. Administering growth hormone to normal volunteers who have been made catabolic by caloric restriction improves the nitrogen balance. The studies described illustrate that administration of somatomedin-C (IGF-I) to catabolic normal volunteers also results in improved nitrogen balance and, unlike growth hormone, does not induce insulin resistance. Growth hormone was anabolic in patients with severe chronic obstructive lung disease and resulted in improved chest wall muscle strength. Both IGF-I and growth hormone have the potential to improve muscle mass and function in patients who are catabolic due to the severity of their underlying disease state.

Introduction

A significant proportion of children and adults who are hospitalized with acute and chronic illnesses show excessive loss of body protein stores. While many of these patients may recover from their illness and regain body mass during the convalescent period, in some patients inability to gain lean body mass increases susceptibility to in-hospital complications (such as nosocomial infections), and in cases of extreme protein wasting may result in severe disability or death. Severe catabolic states prolong hospitalization, increase morbidity and increase rates of in-hospital complications. Since the early 1970s there has been significant interest in reversing catabolic states in hospitalized patients by giving nutritional support therapy. Both intravenous and nasoduodenal tube alimentation methods have had limited success in controlling the rate of catabolism, but these methods often do not produce the accretion of muscle protein that is needed in these patients.

Trials of Growth Hormone in Catabolic States

Moderate Caloric Restriction
Because of the inability of even massive amounts of nutrients to reverse the catabolic state, interest has been raised in the possibility of using growth hormone and/or peptide growth factors as pharmacological agents to treat these disorders. In the 1970s and 80s, studies of growth hormone in catabolic patients were limited by the availability of the hormone. As growth hormone was in scarce supply priority was given to its use in children with short stature, and only a few, limited protocols were undertaken in catabolic patients. In spite of this, two studies in burn patients suggested that an increased anabolic response could be obtained [1, 2]. With the advent of recombinant growth hormone, several trials were initiated in the early 1980s in normal volunteers who had a controlled catabolic state induced by dietary energy restriction. These studies benefitted from a large body of prior research showing that

D.R. Clemmons
Department of Medicine
University of North Carolina
CB-7170 MacNider Building
Chapel Hill, NC 27599–7170 (USA)

0301–0163/92/0388–0037
$ 2.75/0

reduced energy intakes would cause limited, controlled catabolism in normal adults. New tests, such as radioimmunoassay for somatomedin-C (insulin-like growth factor-I; IGF-I), were also important, as they allowed investigators to determine the effectiveness of growth hormone in experimentally-induced catabolism.

IGF-I measurements were deemed particularly useful because IGF-I levels had previously been shown to be dependent on nutrient intake. Studies had shown that if calories or protein were restricted the biosynthetic IGF-I response to endogenous growth hormone secretion was attenuated. Fasting for 9 days resulted in a 70% decrease in IGF-I in adults in spite of an increase in serum growth hormone levels [3]. Merimee et al. showed that total fasting resulted in complete refractoriness of IGF-I secretion to growth hormone administration [4]. In rats this was shown to be due to down-regulation of growth hormone receptors in the liver [5]. Restriction of both protein and energy appear to be the causal factors, as a 66% reduction in protein intake in rats or restriction to 11 kcal/kg in humans severely impairs the IGF-I response to growth hormone [6, 7]. In contrast, energy restriction to 24 kcal/kg does not attenuate the ability of growth hormone to generate an IGF-I response in normal volunteers. Furthermore, in subjects fed the 24 kcal/kg diet, the diet-induced change in nitrogen balance (e.g. a 2.6 g/day loss of nitrogen) was reversed by administering growth hormone. During the first week of receiving growth hormone, patients entered positive nitrogen balance, and a significant response was sustained for an additional 2 weeks [8]. Although the subjects were no longer in positive balance during weeks 2 and 3, their nitrogen balance was statistically significantly less negative than that induced by the caloric restriction alone (e.g. 0.5 g/day versus 2.4 g/day). Therefore, growth hormone was able to attenuate the rate of nitrogen losses significantly in subjects undergoing a modest caloric restriction.

Severe Caloric Restriction

To determine whether the nitrogen-sparing effect of growth hormone was dependent on the level of caloric intake, calories were further restricted to 18 kcal/kg in normal volunteers. Again growth hormone was capable of inducing a significant increase in nitrogen retention in comparison with subjects fed the control diet alone, and this response lasted for approximately 4.5 weeks [9]. After that time, although growth hormone could still induce significant increases in IGF-I, the subjects became refractory to its nitrogen-sparing effects. Direct proof of IGF-I resistance was not established, however. These findings led us to conclude that if growth hormone were to be used alone as an anti-catabolic agent, it would be effective only for limited periods in subjects with this degree of catabolism (i.e. nitrogen losses of 4–5 g/day). This raises the question as to whether subjects with more severe catabolic stresses would respond to growth hormone at all.

To answer this question an additional group of subjects underwent a more severe caloric restriction to 12 kcal/kg ideal body weight (IBW) and growth hormone was administered. In these subjects, as might be predicted, the IGF-I response was no longer maximal and IGF-I levels could only be increased approximately 60% above control compared with a 3.5-fold increase in subjects who were fed a normal caloric intake [10]. Likewise, the improvement in both nitrogen balance and IGF-I responsiveness brought about by administering growth hormone were attenuated much earlier. Significant effects on nitrogen balance occurred for only about 2 weeks, and IGF-I levels had returned to baseline by the end of 3 weeks of growth hormone administration. At that point the subjects were no longer increasing their IGF-I levels in response to growth hormone. Furthermore, even the transient response to growth hormone appeared to be dependent on dietary composition. If calories were supplied primarily as lipid and protein, the volunteers showed no increase in IGF-I and no improvement in nitrogen balance, whereas if 72% of the calories were supplied as carbohydrate there was a transient but significant increase in IGF-I and improvement in nitrogen balance. Hence, a more severe catabolic condition (i.e. nitrogen loss of 6–8 g/day) would result in almost complete refractoriness to the nitrogen-sparing effects of growth hormone. As some catabolic patients may fall in this range, this study suggests that the usefulness of growth hormone may be limited in subjects with extreme catabolic states (>6 g/day nitrogen loss). However, this remains to be proved.

Severe Illness

Studies in subjects with clinically severe illnesses are limited. However, Ward et al. examined the acute effect of growth hormone (6-day study) in postoperative patients who were receiving significant caloric restriction (e.g. 400 kcal/day) [11]. In spite of the significant catabolism induced by recent surgery, growth hormone induced a marked improvement in protein synthesis rates. The response was sustained for the entire 6-day period. The clinical applicability of these findings is limited, however, due to the short duration of the study; based on our findings it is questionable whether this response could be extended for a 2–3-week period.

A second study by Zeigler and colleagues showed that in postoperative patients receiving 1100 kcal/day, a single daily dose of growth hormone, 10 mg/day for 2 weeks, resulted in significant improvement in nitrogen balance [12]. This response to growth hormone is important because these patients had significant catabolism and the response was sustained for 2 weeks. Whether the effect of growth hormone could be sustained beyond this point is unclear. A recent study in patients with severe bacterial sepsis indicates that not all catabolic patients will respond to growth hormone [13]. These patients received growth hormone, 0.05 mg/kg/day for 2 days, but had no improvement in IGF-I or nitrogen balance. This suggests that some patients are refractory to the nitrogen-sparing effects of growth hormone.

We studied a group of severely calorie-restricted volunteers (12 kcal/kg) and administered twice the usual daily dose of growth hormone (0.1 mg/kg IBW) for 3 weeks in order to determine whether or not refractoriness to growth hormone can be overcome by increasing the dose. The higher dose produced a slightly greater increment in nitrogen retention – approximately 0.75 g/day greater than that produced by the usual dose – in normal volunteers who were severely calorically restricted [14]. More importantly the effect was sustained for 4 weeks instead of 2 weeks. This dose of growth hormone also resulted in significant nitrogen retention for about 4 weeks. Therefore, we concluded that doubling the dose of growth hormone resulted in a slight absolute increment in maximal nitrogen retention and a more prolonged period of nitrogen retention.

To determine whether growth hormone had an anabolic effect in cachectic patients suffering from a chronic medical disease we studied the effect of the hormone in patients with chronic obstructive pulmonary disease. Many such patients are less than the ideal body weight in spite of a normal caloric intake, and their weight loss is believed to result in decreased chest wall muscle strength, which further impairs their functional capacity. Seven subjects were placed on a diet containing 35 kcal/kg IBW and 1 g protein [15]. They received this diet for 1 week and then began growth hormone at a dose of 0.05 mg/kg/IBW. Three weeks of growth hormone induced a mean weight gain of 2.2 kg that was not due to fluid retention. Growth hormone also induced a significant improvement in mean nitrogen balance (2.1 g/day) and a 2.4-fold increase in the mean IGF-I concentration. Both of these responses were sustained for the entire 3 weeks of treatment. In addition, the maximum inspiratory force improved significantly from 52 ± 6 to 64 ± 8 cm H_2O. This change was present in six of the seven subjects. No clinically significant toxicity (e.g. oedema or glucose intolerance) was noted. Therefore growth hormone appeared to result not only in nitrogen accretion but also in functional improvement.

Trials of IGF-I in Catabolic States

Because of the problems with toxicity in terms of oedema, arthralgias and worsening glucose tolerance that occur in some patients treated with growth hormone, it may not be possible to treat all catabolic patients. Furthermore, some patients are resistant to the nitrogen-sparing effects of growth hormone [12]. In the latter patients, growth hormone induced no significant increase in IGF-I. To determine whether administering IGF-I would overcome this resistance to growth hormone and would be associated with less toxicity than growth hormone, we undertook a study in normal volunteers who were within 10% of ideal body weight. Our objectives were to discover (a) if IGF-I could promote an anabolic response that was equivalent to a standard dose of growth hormone, (b) if IGF-I was associated with less toxicity than growth hormone, (c) if the known effects of growth hormone on glucose metabolism could be countered with IGF-I treatment, (d) if the anabolic response to IGF-I could be sustained for an equivalent period of time.

Normal volunteers were fed a diet of 20 kcal/kg IBW for 7 days before beginning treatment. They then received daily either a standard dose of growth hormone, 0.05 mg/kg IBW, or an infusion of IGF-I, 12 μg/kg/h for 16 h for 6 days. The IGF-I infusions significantly reduced nitrogen wasting. Nitrogen loss fell from a control value of –3.2 to –0.4 g/day, and this response was sustained for the entire 6-day period. Likewise serum urea nitrogen declined by about 72% in the IGF-I-treated group, and this was maintained during the last 4 days of the 6-day treatment period infusion. Growth hormone induced similar responses in serum urea nitrogen and nitrogen balance, though growth hormone was slightly more effective in terms of nitrogen-promoting capacity at this dose.

The two peptides had opposite effects on glucose metabolism. Specifically, growth hormone increased mean fasting blood glucose by approximately 11% and increased insulin secretion and C-peptide 1.6-fold. In contrast, IGF-I suppressed insulin and C-peptide by approximately 80%, lowered mean fasting blood glucose by 25% and induced significant hypoglycaemia at several points during the infusion [16]. In fact severe hypoglycaemia was a rate-limiting factor for infusion in this study and several subjects had to have their infusion turned off several times to correct severe symptomatic hypoglycaemia and oral glucose had to be administered in some cases.

The findings suggest that IGF-I can mimic the trophic actions of growth hormone if administered in sufficient doses. However, the therapeutic window between maximum nitrogen-retaining effects and induction of severe hypoglycaemia may be limited. We conclude that IGF-I may be most useful in patients with severely impaired glucose tolerance who have a wide therapeutic margin between the systemic IGF-I levels that will promote an anabolic response and those that will induce hypoglycaemia. These studies also suggest that a combination of IGF-I and growth hormone might be needed to induce maximum nitrogen sparing. This would allow administration of higher doses of IGF-I, because growth hormone would be expected to block some of the hypoglycaemia-promoting actions of IGF-I, while IGF-I would attenuate the hyperglycaemic response to growth hormone. It is hoped that this combination can be tested in the near future.

Summary

In summary, both IGF-I and growth hormone appear to be potent anabolic agents in human subjects. Their use may enable us to treat patients with severe catabolic agents more aggressively. The mandate for the future is to begin clinical studies in patients who are catabolic as soon as possible.

References

1 Wilmore DW, Moglan JA, Bristow BF: Anabolic effects of human growth hormone and high caloric feedings following thermal injury. Surg Gynecol Obstet 1974;138:875–884.
2 Soroff HS, Rozin RR, Mooty J: Role of human growth hormone in the response to trauma: Metabolic effects following burns. Ann Surg 1967;166:739–752.
3 Clemmons DR, Klibanski A, Underwood LE, et al: Reduction of plasma immunoreactive somatomedin-C during fasting in humans. J Clin Endocrinol Metab 1981;53:1247–1250.
4 Merimee TJ, Zapf J, Froesch ER: Insulin-like growth factors in fed and fasted states. J Clin Endocrinol Metab 1982;55:999–1002.
5 Maes M, Underwood LE, Ketelslegers JM: Plasma somatomedin-C in fasted and refed rats: Close relationship with changes in liver somatogenic (GH) but not lactogenic (PRL) binding sites. J Endocrinol 1983;97:243–252.
6 Moats-Staats BM, Brady JL, Underwood LE, et al: Dietary protein restriction in artificially reared neonatal rats causes a reduction in insulin-like growth factor I (IGF-I) gene expression. Endocrinology 1984;125:2368–2374.
7 Isley WL, Underwood LE, Clemmons DR: Changes in plasma somatomedin-C in response to ingestion of diets with variable protein and energy content. J Parenter Enteral Nutr 1984; 8:407–411.
8 Clemmons DR, Snyder DK, Williams R, et al: Treatment with growth hormone conserves lean body mass during dietary restriction in obese subjects. J Clin Endocrinol Metab 1987; 64:878–883.
9 Snyder DK, Clemmons DR, Underwood LE: Treatment of obese, diet-restricted subjects with growth hormone for 11 weeks: Effects on anabolism, lipolysis and body composition. J Clin Endocrinol Metab 1988;67:54–61.
10 Snyder DK, Clemmons DR, Underwood LE: Dietary carbohydrate content determines responsiveness to growth hormone in humans. J Clin Endocrinol Metab 1989;69:745–752.
11 Ward HC, Halliday D, Sim AW: Protein and energy metabolism with biosynthetic human growth hormone after gastrointestinal surgery. Ann Surg 1987;206:56–61.
12 Zeigler TR, Young LS, Manson JMcK, et al: Metabolic effects of recombinant human growth hormone in patients receiving parenteral nutrition. Ann Surg 1988;208:6–16.
13 Dahn JJ, Lange MP, Jacobs LA: Insulin-like growth factor 1 production is inhibited in human sepsis. Arch Surg 1988;123:1409–1414.
14 Snyder DK, Underwood LE, Clemmons DR: The anabolic effects of growth hormone in obese diet-restricted subjects are dose dependent. Am J Clin Nutr 1990;52:431–437.
15 Pape GS, Freidman M, Underwood LE, et al: The effect of growth hormone on weight gain and pulmonary function in patients with chronic obstructive lung disease. Chest 1991; 99:1495–1500.
16 Clemmons DR, Smith-Banks A, Celniker AC, et al: Reversal of diet-induced catabolism by infusion of recombinant insulin-like growth factor-I (IGF-I) in humans. J Clin Endocrinol Metab 1992;74.

Horm Res 1992;38(suppl 2):41–43

J.M. Gertner

Department of Pediatrics,
Cornell University Medical College,
New York, NY, USA

Growth Hormone Actions on Fat Distribution and Metabolism

Key Words
Growth hormone
Fat distribution
Metabolism

Abstract
The secretion of growth hormone (GH) and the mass and distribution of body fat are linked through a complex series of interactions. There is increasing evidence that a GH/fat cycle exists and that elements of this cycle may possess regulatory functions. The essential elements of the cycle are: (1) GH-deficient individuals are often obese and lose body fat when they are treated; GH is lipolytic in vitro and causes an acute release of free fatty acids (FFA) when administered in vivo; (3) circulating FFA inhibit the pituitary release of GH by most secretagogues, including growth hormone releasing hormone, and (4) the obese state is characterized by a defect in GH release which can be reversed by weight loss.

Reversible Obesity in Growth Hormone (GH) Deficiency

Severely GH-deficient (and GH-resistant) children have a characteristic 'pudgy' appearance with a predominantly abdominal obesity [1]. In the GH-deficient child undergoing GH replacement therapy, this excess body fat mass reduces [2] and redistributes [3]. In order to determine whether the loss of fatty tissue due to GH therapy is caused by increased lipolysis or decreased lipogenesis, and to compare GH effects at different body sites, we biopsied the abdominal and gluteal fat depots and studied the metabolism of dispersed fat cells freshly obtained from subjects before and during long-term GH replacement. The main effect seen was a decrease in the sensitivity of abdominal fat to the antilipolytic effect of insulin [3]. Interestingly, although it is well known that GH can induce an acute lipolytic response in vivo [4] and in vitro [5], the basal lipolytic rate of fat cells from subjects on GH therapy was unchanged from that of untreated GH-deficient children. In addition, in our study, lipolysis did not change with exposure of the cells to GH in vitro.

Acute Lipolytic Effect of GH

The acute effect of GH on fat metabolism in vivo is quite clear. GH injection causes an acute lipolytic response with consequent increases in serum concentrations of free fatty acids (FFA) and glycerol [6]. The rise in glycerol strongly suggests that the acute increase in FFA is due to lipolysis of existing fat rather than to a sudden reduction in lipid synthesis. The action of GH on fat cells is complex, consisting of at least two components, an early (1–2 h) 'insulin-like' or antilipolytic effect followed by a later more profound 'anti-insulin' lipolytic effect. These two types of action are believed to occur through the interaction of GH with two different types of receptor on the adipocyte [7]. In addition to the direct effect of GH on the rate of hydrolysis of esterified fats, the interaction of GH with the fat cell may alter the sensitivity of the cell to catecholamines, insulin and other agents which influence lipolysis.

J.M. Gertner
Department of Pediatrics
Cornell University Medical College
1300 York Avenue, New York, NY (USA)

FFA Inhibit GH Secretion

The observation that the administration of GH in vivo causes the release of FFA into the circulation is balanced by the finding that FFA can inhibit the release of GH. This action must be effected at the level of the pituitary, because FFA inhibit the somatotrophic response to growth hormone releasing hormone (GHRH) [8]. However the pituitary effect could be indirect with the primary consequence of FFA administration being to increase the release of hypothalamic somatostatin (fig. 1).

The Role of FFA in the Negative Feedback Effect of GH on Its Own Secretion

The administration of exogenous GH to a normal man for up to 3 days inhibits the response of the pituitary to GH secretagogues [9]. These include GHRH, showing that inhibition is at the level of the pituitary. Most authors have assumed that this autoinhibition is mediated by IGF-1. However, our observations led us to doubt whether this was the whole story, because the degree of GH autoinhibition showed no relationship to the induced rise in IGF-1 [10]. Later we [11] and others [12] found that autoinhibition of GH secretion could be induced by a GH infusion over as brief a time as 3 h, probably not enough time to induce the formation of IGF-1 in the pituitary and hypothalamus and certainly too brief a time to see a rise in circulating IGF-1 level.

Our studies led us to hypothesize a homeostatic loop in which GH modulates its own secretion using the serum FFA concentration as a negative feedback messenger. In this scheme, the short-term inhibitory effect exerted by administered GH on endogenous GH release would act via the induced rise in serum FFA concentration. Under the test condition of induced hyperinsulinaemia (to block the rise of FFA), the feedback inhibitory effect of GH infusion on endogenous GH release was no longer seen [13]. However, in a similar attempt to observe the extent of GH autoinhibition during lipolytic blockade, Lanzi et al. [14] successfully used a drug (Acimopox) to block lipolysis and noted a persistence of the autoinhibitory effect of exogenous GH. Thus, they feel that FFA do not play a significant part in the control of pituitary GH release.

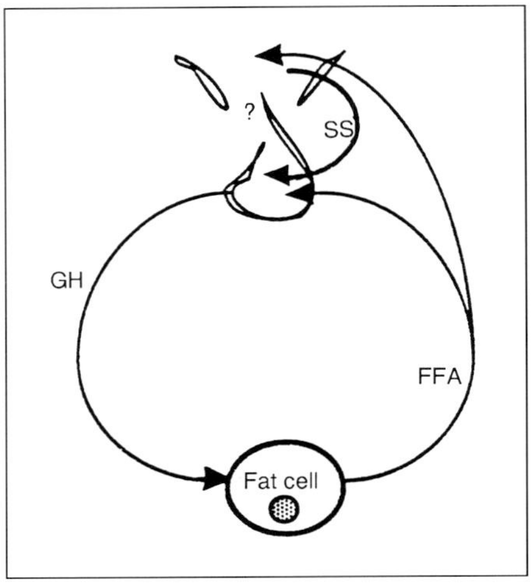

Fig. 1. GH induces lipolysis with consequent increase in circulating FFA. These increased levels in turn suppress somatotrophin secretion, either directly or by promoting the release of hypothalamic somatostatin (SS).

GH Suppressive Effect of the Obese State

Obese subjects secrete much less GH than age-matched controls. This reduced secretion does not appear to be due to altered carbohydrate sensitivity or thyroid function in the obese state [15]. When obese patients were subjected to long-term weight reduction by intestinal surgical techniques, their capacity to secrete GH was restored, indicating that relative GH deficiency is not an innate functional peculiarity of those destined to become obese [16]. The cause of the suppressed state of GH secretion in the obese is not known. Loche and colleagues [17] have suggested that obese children have higher IGF-1 levels than non-obese controls, and this has also been our own observation (unpublished). However, Kelijman and Frohman [18] found that obese adults, with suppressed GH secretion, did not have higher IGF-1 levels than controls and they felt that there were two distinct influences linking the obese state to GH secretion. The first was an acute effect of food intake, seen also in normal weight controls. The second seemed to reflect body weight, in that obese patients who had lost weight secreted more GH in response to GHRH than they did before entering a weight-reduction programme [18].

GH Treatment of Obese Individuals

The twin findings of adipose tissue reduction with exogenous GH replacement to GH-deficient individuals and the secondary GH deficiency of obesity provide the theory behind attempts to treat obesity with administration of GH. The results of such attempts have been inconclusive. One benefit of GH may lie in its capacity to preserve and enhance lean body mass during hypocaloric feeding (dieting) [19]. A recent study has suggested that adipose mass may diminish when obese adults on an ad libitum diet are treated with GH [20]. There is also evidence that GH may promote a net loss of adipose tissue in two other special groups of adults: those with known GH deficiency [21] and the elderly [22]. These topics are currently the focus of very active clinical research.

Conclusion

GH may influence the extent and nature of fat stores; FFA may exert a dynamic effect on GH secretion, and the obese state chronically inhibits GH secretion. Discovering the way in which the elements underlying these phenomena, and other elements not yet discovered, weave into a complete explanation of the link between GH and body fat remains a fascinating challenge. Investigation of the GH/fat cycle will have a significant bearing on two major concerns of paediatric endocrinologists: statural growth and weight control.

References

1 Collipp PJ, Thomas J, Kurti V, et al: Body composition changes in children receiving human growth hormone. Metabolism 1973;22:589–595
2 Parra A, Argote RM, Garcia G, et al: Body composition in hypopituitary dwarfs before and during growth hormone therapy. Metabolism 1979;28:851–857.
3 Rosenbaum M, Gertner JM, Leibel RL: Effects of systemic growth hormone (GH) administration on regional adipose tissue distribution and metabolism in GH-deficient children. J Clin Endocrinol Metab 1989;69:1274–1281.
4 Henneman PH, Forbes AP, Moldawer M, et al: Effects of human growth hormone in man. J Clin Invest 1960;39:1223–1231.
5 Goodman HM, Grichting G: Growth hormone and lipolysis: A reevaluation. Endocrinology 1983;113:697–702.
6 Miller N, Jorgensen JO, Schmitz O, et al: Effects of a growth hormone pulse on total and forearm substrate fluxes in humans. Am J Physiol 1990;258:E86–91.
7 Chipkin SR, Szecowka J, Tai LR, et al: Different growth hormone–receptor interactions mediate insulin-like and lipolytic responses of rat adipose tissue. Endocrinology 1989;125:450–458.
8 Imaki T, Shibasaki T, Shizume K, et al: The effect of free fatty acids on growth hormone (GH)-releasing hormone-mediated GH secretion in man. J Clin Endocrinol Metab 1985;60:290–293.
9 Rosenthal SM, Hulse JA, Kaplan SL, et al: Exogenous growth hormone inhibits growth hormone-releasing factor-induced growth hormone secretion in normal men. J Clin Invest 1986;77:176–180.
10 Nakamoto JM, Gertner JM, Press CM, et al: Suppression of the growth hormone (GH) response to clonidine and GH-releasing hormone by exogenous GH. J Clin Endocrinol Metab 1986;62:822–826.
11 Rosenbaum M, Loche S, Balzano S, et al: Short-term met-hGH infusion inhibits somatotroph response to growth hormone releasing hormone (1–44). Metabolism 1988;37:131–135.
12 Rosenthal SM, Kaplan SL, Grumbach MM: Short term continuous intravenous infusion of growth hormone (GH) inhibits GH-releasing hormone-induced GH secretion: A time-dependent effect. J Clin Endocrinol Metab 1989;68:1101–1105.
13 Rosenbaum M, Fong YM, Hesse DG, et al: Intravenous refeeding blocks growth hormone (GH)-provoked rises in serum free fatty acids and blunting of somatotroph response to GH-releasing hormone in normal men. J Clin Endocrinol Metab 1989;69:310–316.
14 Lanzi R, Pontiroli AE, Monti LD, Monzani M, Pozza G: The growth hormone clamp technique: Inhibition of growth hormone release by growth hormone occurs independently of free fatty acids. Metabolism 1990;39:819–821.
15 Ratzmann KP, Gottschling HD: Abnormal growth hormone response in obesity with normal carbohydrate tolerance and normal thyroid function. Endokrinologie 1978;72:149–154.
16 Williams T, Berelowitz M, Joffe SN, et al: Impaired growth hormone responses to growth hormone-releasing factor in obesity. A pituitary defect reversed with weight reduction. N Engl J Med 1984;311:1403–1407.
17 Loche S, Cappa M, Borrelli P, et al: Reduced growth hormone response to growth hormone-releasing hormone in children with simple obesity: Evidence for somatomedin-C mediated inhibition. Clin Endocrinol 1987;27:145–153.
18 Kelijman M, Frohman LA: Enhanced growth hormone (GH) responsiveness to GH-releasing hormone after dietary manipulation in obese and non-obese subjects. J Clin Endocrinol Metab 1988;66:489–494.
19 Clemmons DR, Snyder DK, Williams R, et al: Growth hormone administration conserves lean body mass during dietary restriction in obese subjects. J Clin Endocrinol Metab 1987;64:878–883.
20 Skaggs SR, Crist DM: Exogenous human growth hormone reduces body fat in obese women. Horm Res 1991;35:19–24.
21 Salomon F, Cuneo RC, Hesp R, et al: The effects of treatment with recombinant human growth hormone on body composition and metabolism in adults with growth hormone deficiency. N Engl J Med 1989;321:1797–1803.
22 Rudman D, Feller AG, Nagraj HS, et al: Effects of human growth hormone in men over 60 years old. N Engl J Med 1990;323:1–6.

Horm Res 1992;38(suppl 2):44–46

M.W. Haymond[a]
F.F. Horber[b]

[a] Nemour's Children's Clinic, University of Florida Health Science Center, Jacksonville, FL, USA;
[b] Medizinische Universitäts-Poliklinik, Inselspital, Bern, Switzerland

The Effects of Human Growth Hormone and Prednisone on Whole Body Estimates of Protein Metabolism

Key Words
Human growth hormone
Prednisone
Leucine
Protein synthesis
Proteolysis, L-[1-^{13}C]leucine
L-[1-^{14}C]leucine

Abstract
Human growth hormone (GH) increases estimates of whole body protein synthesis, but has little effect on the rates of proteolysis either post-absorptively or when absorption occurs during a meal. In contrast to insulin, GH stimulates protein synthesis in skeletal muscle tissue. Prednisone in high doses induces protein catabolism and has been used as a controlled model for catabolic illness. Prednisone increases the rates of proteolysis and amino acid oxidation, but has little effect on estimates of protein synthesis. The administration of high doses of GH together with prednisone prevents the protein catabolic effects of prednisone alone. Thus, GH may provide a new management strategy in patients with significant protein catabolic conditions.

Introduction

Patients with protein catabolic conditions are susceptible to protein malnutrition, which can contribute to the morbidity and mortality of their underlying condition, for example if it results in inadequate tissue healing or compromises their immunocompetency. Patients receiving high dose corticosteroids are known to experience severe losses of body protein pools [1]. In contrast, human growth hormone (GH) is known to cause protein anabolism and growth in GH-deficient children. GH also decreases the nitrogen losses in a variety of protein catabolic conditions, such as fasting and major body burns [2, 3]. Identifying the mechanisms of action of the corticosteroids in the induction of protein wasting and developing therapeutic strategies which might ameliorate or prevent such protein wasting may have major implications in the management of a large number of patients, in whom the only known therapy is the use of high dose corticosteroids.

Protein Metabolism

Early studies of the effects of corticosteroids on whole body protein metabolism utilized nitrogen balance techniques. Such measurements only provide net nitrogen balance information, they do not reveal whether an increase in nitrogen loss is due to an increase in proteolysis, a decrease in protein synthesis or a combination of the two. As a result, little mechanistic information exists about the

M.W. Haymond
Nemour's Children's Clinic
University of Florida Health Science Center
Jacksonville, FL (USA)

0301–0163/92/0388–0044
$ 2.75/0

actions of a particular drug or hormone on whole body protein metabolism.

Isotope dilution techniques, employing labelled leucine, have been used to study the action of cortisol and prednisone on whole body protein metabolism [4, 5]. Infusion of sufficient cortisol to increase the plasma concentrations in the high physiological range, results in an increase in whole body rates of proteolysis within 4–6 h [4]. From in vitro muscle incubation studies, corticosteroids are reported to induce protein wasting, primarily by decreasing the rate of protein synthesis. Oral prednisone at doses of 60 mg/day in normal volunteer adults had little effect on the whole body estimates of protein synthesis. However, it increased the rate of whole body proteolysis and the oxidation of at least one essential amino acid, leucine, in the post-absorptive state. As in the control studies, protein synthesis increased during meal absorption despite significant hyperinsulinaemia, suggesting insulin resistance. However, leucine oxidation continued at rates higher than those of the controls [5]. Thus, in contrast to in vitro incubation studies, corticosteroids in humans appear to cause protein wasting by increasing the rates of proteolysis and oxidation of at least some of the essential amino acids.

GH Effects

In more recent studies, the effects of GH on protein metabolism, in the presence and absence of high dose prednisone, was explored in normal volunteers [6]. GH had no effect on the absorption of labelled leucine nor on its entry into the plasma space. Under both post-absorptive and intracebal conditions, GH significantly increased the estimates of whole body protein synthesis but had no effect on proteolysis. Such studies do not define the site of the increased protein synthesis. However, if the forearm data of Barrett et al. [7] can be extrapolated to these whole body studies, a substantial amount of the increase in protein synthesis observed must have occurred in muscle tissue. The role GH plays in the regulation of splanchnic protein metabolism remains to be determined.

It has been assumed that the mechanism by which GH affects protein synthesis is via the generation of IGF-1. Over the course of several hours of forearm infusion, GH increased estimates of protein synthesis but had little effect on proteolysis. It was observed that the A–V difference in IGF-1 did not change, suggesting that GH may act on muscle directly, or that the IGF-1 was generated intracellularly or there was too little to be quantified by standard A–V stochastic techniques [7]. With the recent availability of rhIGF-1, it is now possible to gain new insights into the mechanism of action of GH and IGF-1. In humans, the infusion of IGF-1, at rates sufficient to cause a decrease in the plasma glucose concentration, results in a decrease in the rate of whole body proteolysis with no increase in estimates of protein synthesis. These results suggest that at rates of IGF-1 infusion sufficient to elicit an insulin-like effect on carbohydrate metabolism, IGF-1 may affect protein metabolism via the insulin receptor and not via the mechanism through which GH elicits its effects. These results have drawn increasing attention to the IGF-1 binding proteins and the role that they may play in directing the effects of IGF-1 to its target tissues.

Conclusion

Although we do not completely understand the mechanism of action of GH, we have demonstrated that GH administration at high doses can prevent the protein catabolic effects of corticosteroid in humans [8]. Whether such use of GH has any practical role in the management of patients receiving high dose corticosteroids remains to be determined. The simultaneous administration of GH and corticosteroids at pharmacological doses resulted in striking insulin resistance and hyperglycaemia, particularly in the intracebal period, despite a significant increase in the plasma IGF-1 concentration [9].

In addition, the effects of GH on the immune system must be clearly established because one of the common uses of high dose corticosteroids is to alter the immune response in patients receiving organ transplants or those with autoimmune diseases. Until the potential risks of such combined therapies have been clearly established, the use of GH in patients receiving high dose corticosteroids must be considered experimental and only used under very carefully defined research conditions.

References

1 Horber FF, Zürcher RM, Herren H, et al: Altered body fat distribution in patients with glucocorticoid treatment and in patients on long-term dialysis. Am J Clin Nutrition 1986; 43:758–769.

2 Clemmons DR, Williams R, Snyder DK, et al: Treatment with growth hormone conserves lean body mass during dietary restriction in obese volunteers. J Clin Endocrinol Metab 1987;64:878–883.

3 Wilmore DW, Maylan JA Jr, Bristow BF, et al: Anabolic effects of growth hormone and high caloric feedings following thermal injury. Surg Gynecol Obstet 1974;138:875–884.

4 Simmons PS, Miles JM, Gerich JE, et al: Increased proteolysis: An effect of increases in plasma cortisol within the physiologic range. J Clin Invest 1984;73:412–420.

5 Beaufrère B, Horber FF, Schwenk WF, et al: Glucocorticosteroids increase leucine oxidation and impair leucine balance in humans. Am J Physiol 1989;257:E712–E721.

6 Horber FF, Haymond MW: Human growth hormone prevents the protein catabolic side effects of prednisone in humans. JCI 1990;86: 265–272.

7 Fryburg DA, Gelfand RA, Barrett EJ: Growth hormone acutely stimulates forearm muscle protein synthesis in normal humans. Am J Physiol 1991;260:E499–E504.

8 Boulware SD, Rennert NJ, Matthews LS, et al: The scope of IGF-1's actions in humans extends to carbohydrate, protein and lipid metabolism. Abstract No. 1613, 73rd Annual Meeting, Endocrine Society, 1991.

9 Horber FF, Horber-Feyder CM, Krayer S, et al: Plasma reciprocal pool specific activity predicts that of intracellular free leucine for protein synthesis. Am J Physiol 1989;257(20): E385–E399.

Horm Res 1992;38(suppl 2):47–49

S. Caprio
D. Boulware
V. Tamborlane

Department of Pediatrics and
The Children's Clinical Research Center,
Yale University School of Medicine,
New Haven, CT, USA

Growth Hormone and Insulin Interactions

Key Words
Puberty
Insulin sensitivity
Insulin secretion
Insulin-dependent diabetes mellitus

Abstract
Insulin and glucose clamp techniques were used to investigate insulin action and insulin secretion during childhood. Preliminary results suggest that growth hormone (GH) therapy leads to changes in glucose, amino acid and insulin responses that are qualitatively similar to those observed during puberty. Furthermore, the insulin resistance normally seen during puberty may be restricted to peripheral glucose metabolism. In patients with Turner's syndrome, data indicate that there is an increase in the glucose-stimulated insulin response which is exaggerated by GH treatment.

Introduction

The onset of puberty is accompanied by a sharp acceleration in linear growth and physical development in healthy children. In addition to increases in sex steroids, elevations in growth hormone (GH) and other growth-promoting factors, such as insulin and insulin-like growth factor 1 (IGF-1) are normally seen during adolescence. While each of these peptides has been shown to have anabolic effects in a variety of in vitro and in vivo systems, the interrelationship between the diverse metabolic actions of these hormones in healthy growing children has not been established. It is also important to determine how such relationships are influenced by diseases (and their treatments) that adversely affect the growth of children.

For the past few years, investigators at the Children's Clinical Research Center, Yale University, USA, have been using sophisticated, but relatively noninvasive, insulin and glucose clamp techniques to examine developmental changes in insulin action and insulin secretion during childhood. Interest in this area originally evolved from studies in children with insulin-dependent diabetes mellitus (IDDM). In our initial investigation, a simplified version of the euglycaemic, hyperinsulinaemic clamp that employed a single dose of insulin (40 mU/m^2 body surface/min) without tracers was used to examine whether puberty-related defects in insulin-stimulated glucose metabolism might explain some of the difficulties in managing the adolescent with IDDM [1]. Surprisingly, the most striking changes in insulin responsiveness were seen in the nondiabetic control subjects. In healthy, non-obese pubertal children, the rate of exogenous glucose required to maintain euglycaemia during the insulin infusion was reduced by a third compared with that in healthy preadolescents and adults [2]. A similar pattern was seen in IDDM patients, but, at each stage of development, the stimulatory effects of insulin were decreased.

Reduction in Insulin Sensitivity

The hormonal change responsible for the development of insulin resistance during puberty has not yet been established. However, a selective effect of either oestrogens or androgens appears unlikely, since insulin sensitivity was reduced to a similar degree in both adolescent boys and girls in our study, and levels of sex steroids would be expected to be even higher in adults, who were more sensi-

S. Caprio
Department of Pediatrics
Yale University School of Medicine
333 Cedar Street, New Haven, CT 06510 (USA)

0301–0163/92/0388–0047
$ 2.75/0

tive to insulin [2]. Furthermore, Yke-Javinen [3] has shown that the rate of insulin-mediated glucose metabolism in normal women (as determined by the clamp technique) is not affected by the phase of the menstrual cycle, despite differences in sex steroid levels. On the other hand, insulin resistance during puberty, as well as the additive effects of IDDM, could be at least partly explained by variations in the concentration of circulating GH. Integrated concentrations of GH increase during normal puberty [4], and GH levels in patients with IDDM are usually higher than those in nondiabetic controls [5]. In our study, the response to insulin was inversely correlated with the mean 24-hour level of GH when all the diabetic and nondiabetic children were considered together [2].

Since the tissue site(s) of the puberty-induced insulin resistance (hepatic vs. peripheral) could not be determined with the simplified clamp, our next study incorporated stable isotope tracer techniques (6,6-$^2H_2$ glucose) and indirect calorimetry before and during sequential 8 and 40 mU/m^2 body surface/min insulin infusions in healthy preadolescents and adolescents [6]. It should be noted that basal rates of glucose turnover were similar in both groups and that insulin-induced suppression of hepatic glucose production was unaffected by puberty. On the other hand, peripheral glucose uptake increased by more than 25% during the low-dose insulin infusion in prepubertal children, but not in the pubertal children. During the high-dose infusion, the increase in insulin-stimulated glucose uptake above basal values was two times greater in prepubertal than in pubertal children [6]. Moreover, this impairment in peripheral glucose uptake was accounted for by a reduction in nonoxidative glucose disposal (storage of glucose); glucose oxidation (measured by indirect calorimetry) rose to a similar extent in both prepubertal and pubertal children. These studies have also provided data which suggest that the insulin resistance normally seen during puberty may be restricted to peripheral glucose metabolism. Both prepubertal and pubertal children were exquisitely sensitive to the suppressive effects of small increments of insulin on the levels of circulating free fatty acid, B-hydroxybutyrate and branched chain amino acids [6].

Compensatory Increase in Insulin Secretion

We next examined whether the puberty-associated reduction in insulin sensitivity is accompanied by compensatory increases in glucose-stimulated insulin secretion in normal children [7]. The hyperglycaemic clamp technique was used to provide a standardized hyperglycaemic stimulus to pancreatic B cells of normal preadolescent and adolescent children, and adults. This study demonstrated that the insulin and C-peptide responses to an equivalent increase in plasma glucose in the upper physiological range (>6.9 mmol/l) were two to three times greater in adolescents, as compared with preadolescents children and adults [7]. This puberty-associated insulin hypersecretion to glucose involved both the first and second phase insulin responses. Moreover, the magnitude of the first and second phase insulin responses was directly correlated with fasting plasma IGF-1 levels (first phase $r=0.68$, $p<0.01$; second phase $r=0.73$, $p<0.01$). A similar correlation between insulin response and IGF-1 was also seen in the adolescent group (first phase $r=0.55$, $p<0.02$; second phase $r=0.62$, $p<0.01$). The first and second phase insulin responses were not correlated with dehydroepiandrosterone sulfate levels in all the children or within the adolescent group alone. Thus, the increased GH secretion that occurs during puberty could account for the insulin resistance, compensatory hyperinsulinaemia, and elevations in IGF-1 concentration that were observed.

In particular, it should be noted that the augmented insulin responses in the healthy teenagers during the hyperglycaemic clamp lead to a greater fall in branched chain and other essential amino acids. These data imply that compensatory hyperinsulinaemia induced by defects in glucose metabolism may serve a beneficial role by amplifying the anabolic effects of insulin on protein metabolism. Such an interpretation is limited, however, since tracer techniques that could provide information about rates of protein turnover were not employed. To rectify this inadequacy, we are now using methods to determine ^{13}C-leucine and deuterated glucose levels in conjunction with clamping techniques, to examine changes in protein and glucose metabolism in GH deficiency before and after therapy with biosynthetic human GH (hGH). Preliminary results suggest that GH therapy leads to changes in glucose, amino acid and insulin responses that are qualitatively similar to those observed during puberty [8].

Turner's Syndrome

Hyperglycaemic clamp studies were also used to assess the effect of GH therapy in girls with Turner's syndrome, since insulin resistance is an early metabolic defect in this disorder [9] that could be exaggerated by GH. Studies were performed in seven patients with Turner's syndrome, before and after 6–12 months of GH therapy, and in seven healthy children [10]. Fasting plasma insulin levels were comparable in controls and patients before therapy, but increased significantly in the patients with Turner's syndrome after GH treatment. Despite identical glucose increments during the glucose clamp procedure (>6.9 mmol/l above baseline), both the first and second phase insulin responses were significantly greater in the patients with Turner's syndrome. Moreover, the hyperinsulinaemic responses to glucose were markedly exaggerated in the patients with Turner's syndrome following GH therapy, reaching values (first phase 474 + 100 pmol/l and second phase 826 + 100 pmol/l, $p<0.02$ vs. pretreatment) that were almost three times higher than in controls ($p<0.001$). Nevertheless, the rate of insulin-stimulated glucose metabolism during the last 60 min of the clamp was similar in all three studies. Glycosylated haemoglobin, total cholesterol and blood pressure remained normal after GH therapy. These data indicate that glucose-stimulated insulin responses are increased in patients with Turner's syndrome, and that these alterations are further exaggerated by GH treatment. Furthermore, these hyperinsulinaemic responses appear to compensate for reductions in insulin sensitivity.

Acute Metabolic Effects of GH

The acute metabolic effects of GH in the absence of compensatory hyperinsulinaemia were examined in 14 well controlled, insulin-pump treated IDDM patients [11]. GH was given in 100 μg intravenous pulses hourly for 21–45 h, while insulin doses and meals were kept constant [11]. Mean 24-h levels of GH doubled, but levels of free insulin and glucagon were unaffected. Fasting plasma glucose levels rose from 5.7 + 0.6 to 11.3 + 1.0 mmol/l, due mainly to a marked stimulation of hepatic glucose production. Even more surprisingly, levels of circulating amino acids, free fatty acids and ketones were also increased. These data suggest that increases in GH, in the absence of compensatory hyperinsulinaemia, can have catabolic rather than anabolic effects. Therefore, to evaluate fully the metabolic consequences of altering GH levels in health and disease in childhood, physiological adaptations in insulin secretion and insulin action must be taken into account.

References

1 Diabetes Control and Complications Trial Research Group: The diabetes control and complications trial: Results of the feasibility study (phase II). Diabetes Care 1987;10:1–19.

2 Amiel SA, Sherwin RS, Simonson DC, et al: Impaired insulin action in puberty. A contributing factor to poor glycemic control in adolescents with diabetes. N Engl J Med 1986;315:215–219.

3 Yke-Javinen H: Insulin sensitivity during the menstrual cycle. J Clin Endocrinol Metab 1984;59:350–353.

4 Miller JD, Tannerbaum GS, Colle E, et al: Daytime pulsatile growth hormone secretion during childhood and adolescence. J Clin Endocrinol Metab 1982;55:989–994.

5 Horner JM, Kemp SF, Hintz RL: Growth hormone and somatomedin in insulin-dependent diabetes mellitus. J Clin Endocrinol Metab 1981;53:1148–1153.

6 Amiel SA, Caprio S, Sherwin RS, et al: Insulin resistance of puberty: A defect restricted to peripheral glucose metabolism. J Clin Endocrinol Metab 1991;72:277–282.

7 Caprio S, Plewe G, Diamond MP, et al: Increased insulin secretion in puberty: A compensatory response to reductions in insulin sensitivity. J Pediatr 1989;963–967.

8 Boulware SD, Caprio S, Jones TW, et al: Metabolic alterations induced by growth hormone treatment mirror changes during normal adolescence. Pediatr Res 1990;27:72A.

9 Caprio S, Boulware SD, Diamond M, et al: Insulin resistance: An early metabolic effect of Turner syndrome. J Clin Endocrinol Metab 1991;72:832–836.

10 Caprio S, Press CM, Sherwin RS, et al: Insulin resistance and hyperinsulinemia: Characteristic features of Turner syndrome. Pediatric Res 1988;23:237A.

11 Press CM, Tamborlane WV, Sherwin RS: Importance of raised growth hormone levels in mediating the metabolic derangements of diabetes. N Engl J Med 1984;310:810–815.

Horm Res 1992;38(suppl 2):50

P.C. Sizonenko

Introduction

During the Symposium of Paediatric Endocrinology organized in Telf, Austria, a workshop was devoted to sexual differentiation. Recent findings, which have increased our understanding of the mechanisms of sexual differentiation in man, were presented and discussed. Sex differentiation occurs at four different levels: (1) the sex chromosomes; that is, the Y chromosome is the acting chromosome for male sex, two X chromosomes being necessary for full development of the ovary; (2) the development of the fetal gonads; (3) the development and the differentiation of the sex organs and the related secondary structures; (4) the sexual differentiation of the brain.

Dr J.R. Hawkins reported important progress in the isolation and characterization of the gene responsible for the testis, named the SRY gene (the sex-determining region of the Y chromosome). The gene was cloned both in the mouse and in man, and contains a DNA binding motif. Mutations of the SRY gene have also been found in the genomes of XY females. Mutations of several types were found: these include point mutations or mutations in the DNA binding domain, which are conditionally sex reversing.

Gonadal differentiation has been investigated, mainly using molecular biology techniques. Dr R. Voutilainen presented data on the expression of the different genes coding for enzyme activities in the testis and the ovary. A surprising observation was that the ovary is rather quiescent during fetal development. Maleness is mainly expressed by the secretion of testosterone, which enables the genitalia to develop as male sexual organs. In addition, Dr Voutilainen showed that the fetal pituitary is already active and secreting gonadotropins in utero. In addition, Dr N. Josso has studied the secretion of anti-Müllerian hormone by the Sertoli cells of the testis. She advocated the measurement of anti-Müllerian hormone by radioimmunoassay (RIA) for the diagnosis of anorchidism or intersex, in which the presence of the testes is sought.

Dr I.A. Hughes and Dr D. Aarskog then dealt with the clinical aspects of male pseudohermaphroditism and the combination of intersex with dysmorphology. The clinical approach for the diagnosis and management of these conditions was presented and, in particular, the responsiveness of genital tissue to androgens in androgen-insensitivity syndromes.

Finally, Dr D.F. Swaab presented evidence both in animals and in man for the presence of sex differences in the functional and structural architecture of the brain. A sexually dysmorphic nucleus has been described, which is twice as large in men as in women; a similar sex difference was observed in some hypothalamic nuclei. In homosexuals, the volume and number of cells in this nucleus was found to be twice as large as that in a heterosexual control group. The functional implications of such differences remain unclear.

This symposium was extremely rewarding, as all the speakers presented their own new data, most of which was quite recent. Publication of these presentations is, therefore, particularly worthwhile.

Horm Res 1992;38(suppl 2):51–61

D.F. Swaab[a]
L.J.G. Gooren[b]
M.A. Hofman[a]

[a] Netherlands Institute for Brain Research, Amsterdam;
[b] Department of Endocrinology, Free University, Amsterdam, The Netherlands

Gender and Sexual Orientation in Relation to Hypothalamic Structures

Key Words
Hypothalamus
Sexual orientation
Gender

Abstract
Animal experiments have provided evidence for the presence of sex differences from the synaptic level up to behaviour. Although sex differences in the human brain may have been presumed implicitly since the days of Aristotle, research on the presence of functional and structural sex differences of the human brain started only relatively recently. The most conspicuous sex difference in the mammalian brain was described by Gorski et al. [1978] in the preoptic area (POA) of the rat hypothalamus. We found that the volume of a putative homologue of this sexually dimorphic nucleus (SDN) in the adult human hypothalamus was more than twice as large in men as in women and contained about twice as many cells. Recently a similar sex difference and volume has been described for the human bed nucleus of the stria terminalis and 'interstitial nuclei of the hypothalamus' (INAH). Sexual differentiation of the hypothalamus was generally believed to take place between 4 and 7 months of gestation. A life span study on the SDN of more than 100 subjects revealed, however, that only after the age of 2–4 years postnatally sexual differentiation becomes manifest by a decrease in volume and cell number in the female SDN. If sexual differentiation of the brain indeed takes place postnatally, not only chemical and hormonal factors may influence this process but also social factors.

A prominent theory on the development of sexual orientation is that it develops as a result of an interaction between the developing brain and sex hormones. According to Dörner's hypothesis, male homosexuals have a female differentiation of the hypothalamus. This hypothesis was not supported by our observations on the SDN. Neither the SDN volume nor the cell number in the hypothalamus of homosexual men differed from that of heterosexual men. However, a difference in SCN cell number was observed in relation to sexual orientation. The volume and cell number of the SCN of homosexual men was twice as large as that of a reference group. During development, the SCN volume and cell counts reach peak values around 13–16 months after birth. At this age the SCN contains about the same number of cells as the SCN of adult male homosexuals, whereas in the reference group the cell numbers subsequently decline to the adult value, which is about 35% of the peak value. The observation that an SCN similarly enlarged as that observed in homosexual men was present in a woman with Prader-Willi syndrome, a congenital LHRH deficiency in which sex hormones are very low, suggests that at some stage of brain development the interaction with sex hormones might be essential for the programmed SCN cell death.

In conclusion, marked sex differences in the human hypothalamus are found in the SDN and BST, and an enlarged SCN is present in homosexual men. The functional implications of such differences in relation to gender and sexual orientation are, however, far from clear at the moment.

D.F. Swaab
Netherlands Institute for Brain Research
Meibergdreef 33
NL–1105 AZ Amsterdam ZO (The Netherlands)

0301–0163/92/0388–0051
$ 2.75/0

Introduction

Between 4 years of age and puberty we become aware of our gender identity (i.e. being a boy or a girl) and our sexual orientation (i.e. being heterosexual or homosexual). All possible combinations of gender identity and forms of sexual orientation have been described. Some combinations are less valued than others by society, and because of this some have tried to change gender identity or sexual orientation; though with little success. This is probably because gender identity and sexual orientation are fixed in the brain. The present paper gives some recent evidence for this concept.

Sexual Differentiation of the Human Hypothalamus

Following observations in many mammalian species, one is inclined to believe that the human brain undergoes sexual differentiation during its development, due to an organizing effect of sex hormones. However, the stage of development at which sex steroids determine sexual differentiation of the human brain is unknown, as are the exact functional implications of such hormonal actions in relation to gender and sexual orientation. There are three sex-dimorphic peaks in gonadal hormone levels which could be of importance for these processes: during the first half of gestation, when the genitalia are formed [1]; in the perinatal period; and during puberty [2]. Also, total brain weight in adults is sexually dimorphic [3]. The brain area thought to be the primary substrate of sex differences in reproduction, gender identity and sexual orientation is the hypothalamus [4–6]. The supposition that structural sexual differentiation of the human hypothalamus takes place between 4 and 7 months of gestation [7] was based on the observations that: (1) during this period various hypothalamic cell groups (the supraoptic, ventromedial and paraventricular nucleus) can be distinguished histologically (although sex differences in these nuclei were not reported); and (2) the matrix layer surrounding the third ventricle, in which the cells are formed, has disappeared by 7 months of gestation. Later it became clear that cell death rather than cell division may be the most important mechanism in the sexual differentiation of the nervous system [8, 9].

Sexually Dimorphic Nucleus

The sexually dimorphic nucleus (SDN) of the preoptic area of the hypothalamus, as first described in the rat by Gorski et al. [10], is the most conspicuous morphological sex difference in the mammalian brain. The cell group, which is 3–8 times larger in male rats than in female rats (fig. 1), has such a clear cytoarchitectonic sex difference that it can be seen with the naked eye in Nissl-stained sections. Lesions of the SDN affect masculine components of sexual behaviour in the rat, and SDN size is correlated to male sexual activity [11–13]. On the other hand, the changes in sexual behaviour following SDN lesions are so modest that the major function of the SDN has probably not yet been revealed.

Human SDN

We have found an SDN in the preoptic area of the human hypothalamus that is (judging by its localization and cytoarchitecture) probably homologous to that in the rat [14], although proof for such homology, on the basis of transmitter content, afferents and efferents is lacking (fig. 2). Morphometric analysis of the human SDN revealed that the volume is more than twice as large in adult men as in women, and contains approximately twice as many cells in men (fig. 3). The human SDN corresponds to the intermediate nucleus described by Braak and Braak [16] and to the intermediate lateral hypothalamic area described by Brockhaus [17] and Feremutsch [18]. However, it does not correspond with the intermediate nucleus of an earlier paper of Feremutsch [19], who described the islands of neurosecretory cells between the supraoptic and paraventricular nucleus (SON, PVN) by this name. Because of this confusion, we will use the name SDN in the present paper.

The sex difference which we observed in the SDN was not present in other hypothalamic nuclei (fig. 1). The magnitude of the sex difference did not remain constant throughout adulthood, but depended on age (fig. 3). In males, a major reduction in SDN cell number was observed between the age of 50 and 60 years, so that the sex difference became smaller. In females over 70 years of age, cell death was found to be more prominent than in males, dropping to values which were only 10–15% of the cell number found in early childhood. Thus, the sex difference in SDN increases again in old people [15]. This sex difference in the pattern of ageing, and the fact that sexual differentiation in the human SDN only occurs after the fourth year of age [9] might explain why Allen et al. [20], who had a sample of human adults biased for age, did not find a significant sex difference in the size of the SDN (which they called interstitial nucleus of the anterior hypothalamus 1 (INAH-1). In that study [20], 40% of the adult subjects came from the age group in which the SDN sex difference is minimal, compared with 29% in our study [15]. Moreover, the age group of elderly subjects (over 70 years of age) was under-repre-

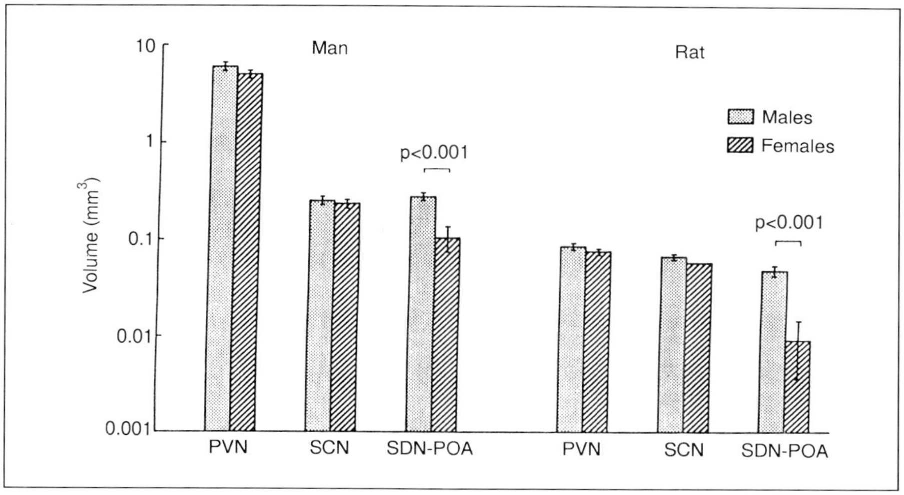

Fig. 1. Volumes of hypothalamic regions in young adult rats (2–5.5 months) and in man (20–40 years). Values represent the mean volume (±SEM) from one hemisphere. The variance of the suprachiasmatic nucleus (SCN) volume in female rats could not be determined. The sexual differences in the volume of the sexually dimorphic nucleus in the preoptic area of the hypothalamus (SDN-POA) were statistically significant, both in man and in the rat. (From Hofman and Swaab [15] with permission.)

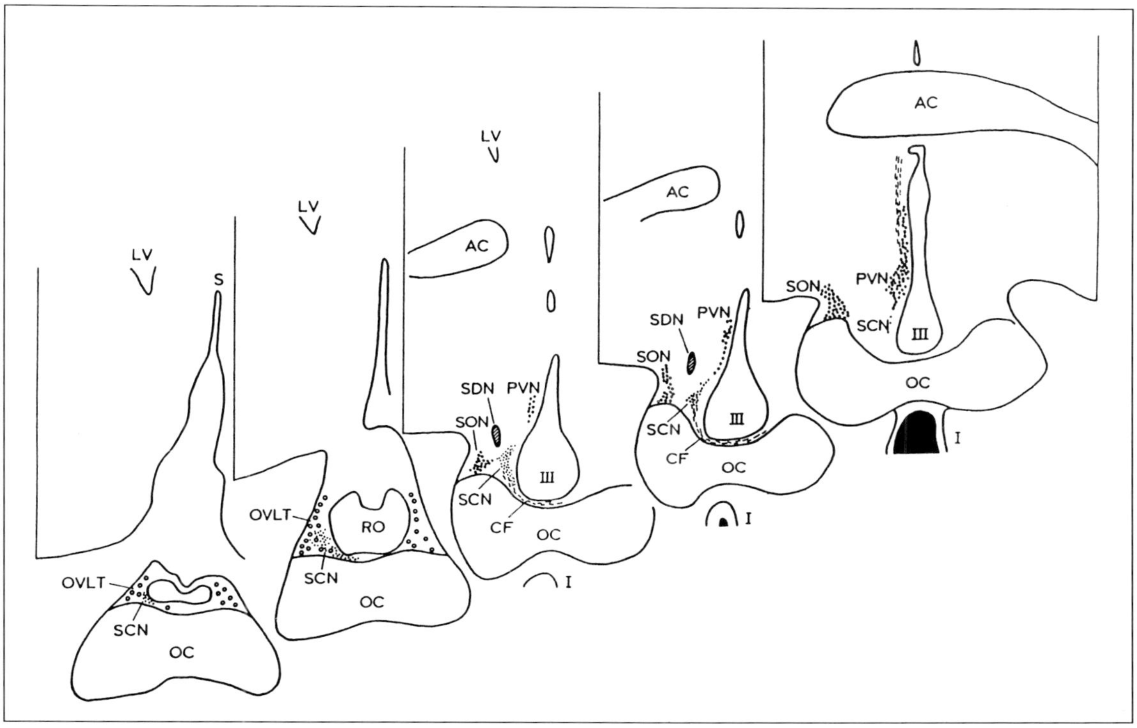

Fig. 2. Topography of the sexually dimorphic nucleus (SDN) in the preoptic area of the human hypothalamus. Third ventricle, III; anterior commissure, AC; infundibulum, I; lateral ventricle, LV; optic chiasm, OC; organum vasculosum of the lamina terminalis, OVLT; recessus opticus, RO; septum, S; suprachiasmatic nucleus, SCN; paraventricular nucleus, PVN; supraoptic nucleus, SON; commissural fibres of the suprachiasmatic nucleus, CF. (From Swaab and Fliers [14] with permission; copyright 1985 by the AAAS.)

sented in Allen's study [20]: 20% compared with 37.5% in the case of a proportional distribution of all ages. In our study, 32% of the subjects belonged to this old age group. It seems thus likely that Allen et al. [20] were unable to establish a sex difference in the INAH-1 (i.e. SDN) because they used a biased sample. A further argument for this assumption is that, if we [15] had studied only subjects of the age distribution of Allen's study, the sex difference in SDN volume would have been reduced from 2 to only 1.4 times, and this difference would not have been statistically significant.

Moreover, the sex difference in the SDN emerges only between the ages of 4 years and puberty [9]; therefore the brains of the 5-year-old boy and 4-year-old girl (she indeed had by far the largest volume of the entire series of female INAH-1) also produced a substantial bias in the Allen et al. [20] study material. However, the age distribution does not explain why LeVay [21] could not find a sex difference in the volume of INAH-1. However, cell numbers were not determined by this author.

Other Sexually Dimorphic Nuclei

Allen et al. [20] described two other cell groups (INAH-2 and -3) in the preoptic-anterior hypothalamic area that were larger in the male brain than in the female brain. LeVay [21] could not confirm the sex difference in INAH-2, but did find a difference in INAH-3. As immunocytochemistry was not performed, it is not clear whether the nuclei have to be considered as islands of the PVN or as separate anatomical entities. In addition, cell counts of the INAHs in the two sexes are lacking.

A clear sex difference was described by Allen and Gorski [22] in what they called the 'darkly staining posteromedial component of the bed nucleus of the stria terminalis (BNST-dspm)', an area in which the volume was found to be 2.5 times larger in males than in females. However, cell counts were not performed in this study, and therefore these findings remain preliminary.

The suprachiasmatic nucleus (SCN) stained with vasopressin as a marker, showed a sex difference in shape [23]. The shape of the SCN was elongated in women and more spherical in men. However, in this study no significant sex difference was observed in either volume, vasopressin cell number or total cell number of the SCN. It is not known whether this sex difference in shape correlates with sex differences in SCN afferent or efferent connections.

Only a few human brain structures in the two sexes have been investigated morphometrically, but as there is a sex difference in the relative size of the human brain [3], we expect that many more sex differences have yet to be revealed.

Development of the Human SDN

In mid-pregnancy the SDN can be distinguished in the human fetal brain [9, 24]. Yet the SDN cell number (fig. 4) and volume at term birth are only 22% and 18%, respectively, of the values found between 2 and 4 years of postnatal age. In the second half of gestation and during the first postnatal years there is no significant sex difference in the size of the SDN. During the first postnatal years the SDN cell number rapidly increases in both boys and girls up to the age of 2–4 years postnatally. Only after this age does the human SDN differentiate according to sex, due to a decrease in both SDN volume and cell number in women, whereas in men these parameters remain unaltered up to the age of about 50 years [9]. Our results do not support the proposition that gonadal hormones stimulate mitotic formation, migration or aggregation of SDN cells during the fetal or perinatal period. In mid-gestation and perinatally the levels of sex hormones are much higher in boys than in girls [1, 2]. Yet, the SDN size and cell number show the same magnitude in boys and girls up to the age of 2–4 years. The surprisingly late postnatal sexual differentiation of the human hypothalamus is in agreement with the observation that neither oestrogen, androgen nor progestin receptors were found in the human fetal brain at mid-gestation [25]. The sex difference in the volume of the BNST-dspm seems to occur only in adulthood, though there is reason for caution. The sample size of subjects between 10 and 20 years of age was small in the Allen and Gorski study [22]. Together, these data support, however, the notion that sexual differentiation of the human hypothalamus takes place after the

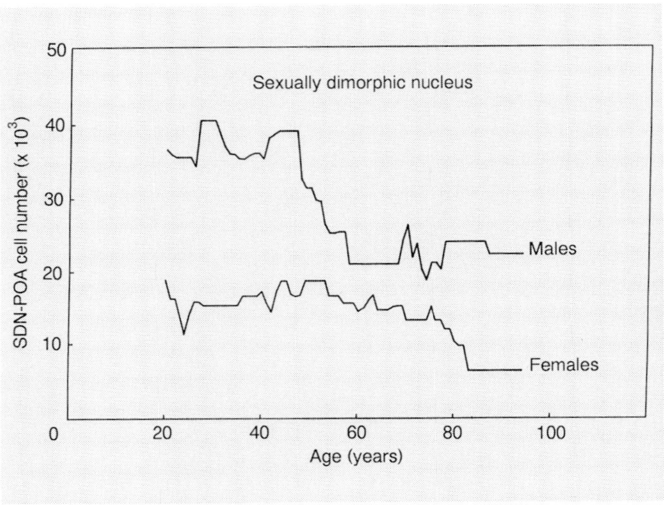

Fig. 3. Age-related changes in the total cell number of the sexually dimorphic nucleus (SDN) of the preoptic area (POA) in the human hypothalamus. The general trend in the data is enhanced by using smoothed growth curves. Note that in males SDN-POA cell number steeply declines between the age of 50 and 60 years, whereas in females, from the age of about 50 years, a more gradual cell loss is observed, which continues until old age. These growth curves demonstrate that the reduction in cell number in the human SDN-POA in senescence is a non-linear, sex-dependent process. (From Hofman and Swaab [15] with permission.)

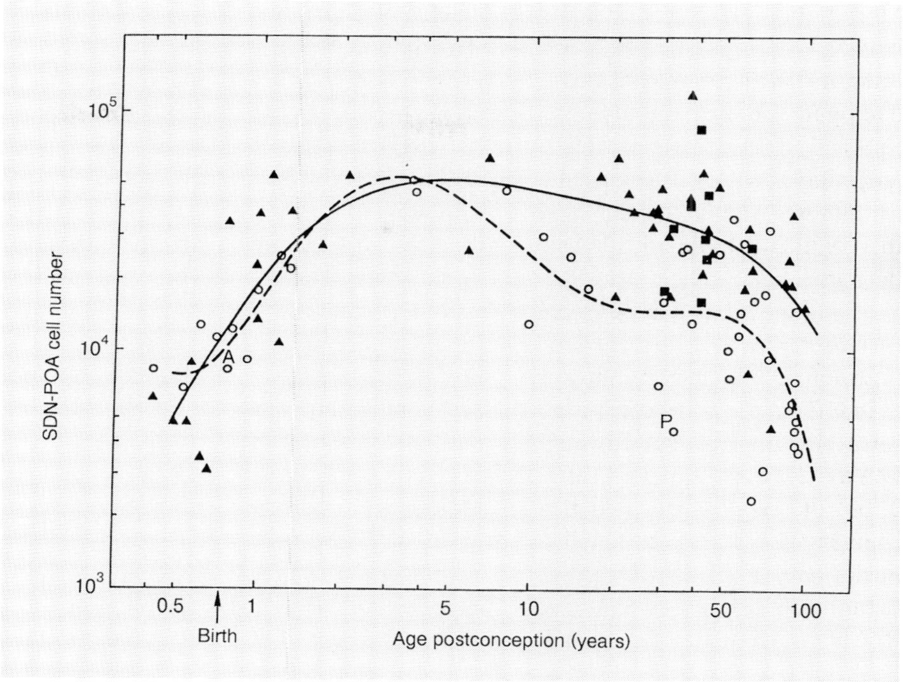

Fig. 4. Development and sexual differentiation of the human sexually dimorphic nucleus (SDN) of the preoptic area (POA) of the hypothalamus. Log-log scale. Note that at the moment of birth the SDN is equally small in boys (▲) and girls (○) and contains only about 20% of the cell number found at 2–4 years of age. The SDN cell number of a female neonate with a pituitary aplasia (A) is fully within the range of other neonates. Cell numbers reach a peak value at approximately 2–4 years postnatally, after which sexual differentiation occurs in the SDN. The cell number in the SDN of women decreases, whereas the cell number in men remains approximately unchanged until the age of 50 years. In women, cell number decreases for the second time after the age of about 60 years, following a period of relative stability, dropping to values which are only 10–15% of the cell numbers found at 2 years postnatally. Note that in men the reduction in cell number in senescence is less dramatic. The largest discrepancy in cell number between men and women is found at approximately 30 years of age and in people older than 80 years, whereas sexual dimorphism in the SDN cell number is least around the age of 60 years. The SDN cell number in homosexual men (■) does not differ from that in the male reference group. The cell number of the SDN of a woman with Prader-Willi syndrome (P) is small. The curves are quintic polynomial functions fitted to the original data for males (drawn line) and females (dashed line). (Adapted from Swaab and Hofman [9] with permission.)

perinatal period and before adulthood, rather than during mid-gestation. This, and our observation that sexual differentiation of the human SDN does not take place earlier than 4 years postnatally, calls for a re-evaluation of the possible relationship between the sex dimorphism of the SDN and the perinatal testosterone peak in boys, which lasts only some 90 days [26]. It is possible that the perinatal testosterone peak promotes cell survival a few years later by preventing the 'programmed' cell death which normally occurs in the female SDN. A similar mechanism is supposed to take place in rat spinal cord neurones of the bulbocavernosus musculature [8].

In addition, one may speculate that not only hormones, but also other chemical compounds and social factors, such as stress, might be involved in sexual differentiation of the brain in this period (compare [9, 27]). A case history of a 20-year-old man who had suffered a complete loss of testes at birth, showed a lack of sequelae in terms of gender identity, gender role and sexual functioning [28]. This observation may support the idea that factors other than androgens may be involved in sexual differentiation of the brain, or that the hormonal factors in the development of gender and sexual orientation exert their effects before birth.

SDN Development and Sex Hormones

Regarding the possible involvement of sex hormones in SDN development in humans, few data are available. Sources of information are the 'experiments of nature and medicine'. A child that died, perinatally, of a pituitary aplasia had a normal sized SDN (fig. 4; [9]). It is of interest, though, that a 30-year-old woman with Prader-Willi syndrome, which is characterized by a congenital deficiency in luteinizing hormone-releasing hormone (LHRH) and sex hormones [29], had a small SDN (fig. 4; [9]). A small SDN was also found in a 57-year-old man with Klinefelter's syndrome, a condition that is characterized by a deficiency in androgen production [Swaab, unpublished results]. Whether these anomalies invariably lead to a smaller SDN in adulthood deserves further investigation. It must be noted that women normally do not have significant elevations of sex steroid levels in early development and that the endocrine differences of Klinefelter patients only become apparent in early puberty [30]. It is, therefore, also conceivable that the genetic anomalies have had an influence on the size of the SDN rather than sex steroid levels during development. However, arguing against this is the fact that in two such different conditions as Klinefelter's and Prader-Willi's syndrome the same anomalies were observed. One might also wonder whether these observations have implications for the development of sexual orientation. Vogt [31] did not find an indication for a higher incidence of homosexuality in his sample of 30 (46, XXY) Klinefelter patients. However, it must be noted that 15 men in his sample were sexually less active than normal males. This prevents any firm conclusion as to the sexual orientation of these subjects.

The Human Hypothalamus, Sexual Orientation and Gender Identity

We had the opportunity to study the structure of the anterior hypothalamus in relation to sexual orientation, and investigated 34 subjects. Eighteen male subjects, 22–74 years of age, whose sexual orientation was generally not known, served as a reference group. The homosexual male group consisted of 10 non-demented AIDS subjects aged 25–43 years. Six non-demented heterosexuals (4 males, 2 females aged 21–73 years) who had also died of AIDS served as a control group. Two areas of the hypothalamus were studied: the SDN and the suprachiasmatic nucleus (SCN). The SCN is considered to be the principal component of the biological clock generating and coordinating hormonal, physiological and behavioural circadian rhythms [32–34]. In addition, the SCN is thought to be involved in reproduction, at least in laboratory animals [35, 36]. The main results were as follows: cell numbers in the SDN of the reference group, the male homosexuals and the heterosexual subjects did not differ. However, the SCN volume in homosexual men was 1.7 times as large as that of the reference group of male subjects and contained 2.1 times as many cells (fig. 5).

The SDN and Sexual Orientation

A prominent theory of sexual orientation is that it develops as a result of an interaction between the developing brain and sex hormones [6, 38–40]. A multitude of factors, such as maternal stress [11, 39, 41 but compare 42, 43] and chemicals [44] are thought to influence the process of sexual differentiation of the brain and sexual orientation. According to Dörner's hypothesis, male homosexuals have a female differentiation of the hypothalamus. This hypothesis was based solely on indirect evidence; the demonstration of a positive feedback of luteinizing hormone (LH) secretion in some homosexual men following injection of oestrogens [6, 45]. However, according to Gooren [46, 47], this phenomenon is probably related to changes in testicular function rather than to sexual orientation, and in his studies it could be demonstrated as often in homosexual as in heterosexual men. Furthermore, it could be shown that the same person was able to produce a negative and a positive oestrogen feedback effect, depending on the hormonal milieu. This demonstrated that it is not the organization of the hypothalamic-pituitary unit that determines the occurrence of a positive or negative oestrogen feedback. Also, it is not certain whether the rise in LH following oestrogen administration that Dörner [45] and Gladue et al. [6] observed, met the stringent endocrine criteria of a positive oestrogen feedback effect [48]. Dörner's hypothesis concerning sexual orientation became testable when we found that the SDN of the preoptic area of the human hypothalamus contains twice as many cells in men as in women [9, 14, 15]. In contrast to this hypothesis, neither the SDN volume nor the cell number in the hypothalamus of homosexual men (who died of AIDS) differed from that of the male reference group in the same age range (fig. 5; [9]). More recent data (fig. 5) confirmed and extended this observation with a heterosexual control group of subjects also suffering from AIDS [37]. The fact that no difference in SDN cell number was observed between homosexual and heterosexual men who died of AIDS refutes the global formulation of Dörner's hypothesis that male homosexuals have 'a female hypothalamus'.

The SCN and Sexual Orientation

The observation that the SCN in homosexual men contains 2.1 times as many cells as the SCN of the reference group (fig. 5; [37]) implies that the difference in SCN vol-

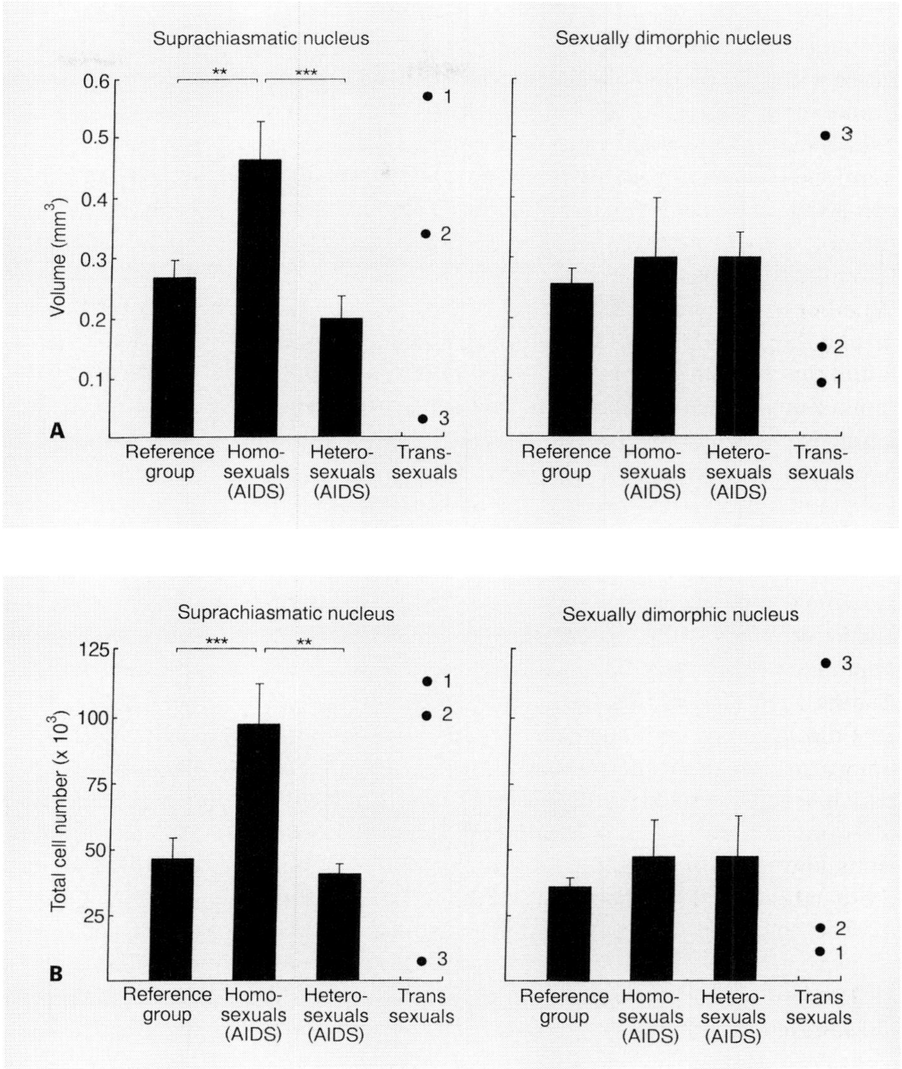

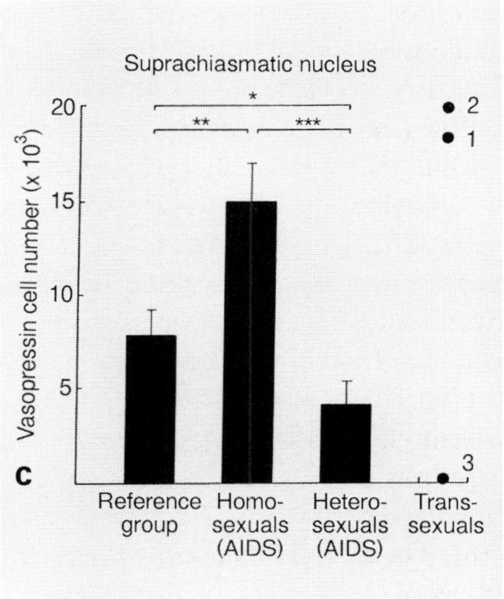

Fig. 5. A Volume of the human suprachiasmatic nucleus (SCN) and sexually dimorphic nucleus (SDN) as measured in four groups of adult subjects: (1) a male reference group (n = 18); (2) male homosexuals who died of AIDS (n = 10); (3) heterosexuals who died of AIDS (n = 6; 4 males and 2 females), and (4) three male-to-female transsexuals (numbers refer to T1–T3 in table 1). The values are medians and standard deviations. The differences in the volume of the SCN between homosexuals and the subjects from both other groups are statistically significant (Kruskal-Wallis multiple comparison test, *$p<0.05$; **$p<0.01$; ***$p<0.001$). Note that none of the parameters measured in the SDN (fig. 5A, B) showed significant differences among the three groups (p always >0.4). **B** Total number of cells in the human SCN and SDN. The SCN in homosexual men contains 2.1 times as many cells as in the reference group of male subjects and 2.4 times as many cells as the SCN in heterosexual AIDS patients. **C** The number of vasopressin (VP) neurones in the human SCN (the human SDN does not contain VP-producing cells). The SCN in homosexual men contains, on average, 1.9 times as many VP-producing neurones as the reference group of male subjects and 3.6 times as many VP neurones as the SCN in heterosexual AIDS patients. Notice that the SCN of heterosexual individuals who died of AIDS contains less VP cells than the subjects from the reference group. In the right-hand column of each figure, the individual values of three transsexual patients (T1–T3) are given. Note that 1 and 2 have a large SCN and a small SDN and that 3 has a small SCN and a large SDN. For clinical details see table 1. (Adapted from Swaab and Hofman [37] with permission.)

ume can not be attributed to differences in shrinkage of hypothalamic tissue during the histological procedure. However, the difference in SCN cell number in relation to sexual orientation can not be directly related to sexual differentiation of the brain since no differences in SCN volume or cell number were found between males and females [23, 49]. The possibility can not be excluded that sex hormone levels during brain development play some part in this phenomenon.

The association between a large SCN (and in particular an increase in the number of neurones) and male homosexuality raises a number of questions about the way this difference might have developed. It appears very unlikely that homosexual behaviour would increase the neuronal number in any brain structure. The nerve cells of the SCN are postmitotic from a few years of age onwards, if not earlier [50]. However, an increase in stainability of vasopressin neurones due to homosexual behaviour can not be excluded. Yet the developmental course of SCN cell numbers [50] suggests that the explanation for the large SCN in homosexual men may be found in the early processes of brain development. At birth, the SCN contains only 13–20% of the adult number of vasopressin and total cells, but in the postnatal period development is rapid. Cell counts reach a peak at 13–16 months after birth [50]. The SCN cell numbers found in adult homosexual men were of the same order of magnitude as found at 13–16 months postnatally. The normal pattern is that the vasopressin and total cell numbers subsequently decline to the adult value of approximately 35% of the peak values. In homosexual men, therefore, this programmed postnatal cell death in the SCN seems to have been reduced. The observation that a similarly enlarged SCN was present in a woman with Prader-Willi syndrome [36], a congenital LHRH deficiency in which sex hormone levels are very low [29] suggests that the interaction with sex hormones at some stage of development might be relevant for the programmed SCN cell death (however, see the caveat earlier in this text). The possibility of sex hormones playing some role in SCN development is reinforced by an observation of Södersten et al. [35]. They showed that the amplitude of the circadian rhythm in sexual behaviour, of which the SCN is the substrate, is enhanced by anti-oestrogen treatment of the neonatal animal. This observation and the large SCN in Prader-Willi syndrome [36] make it more likely that a larger SCN, as reported here for homosexual men, may relate to a difference in the interaction with sex hormones during development. This possibility should be tested in animal experiments and further explored in human material.

One might argue that the present finding of an enlarged SCN in male homosexuals who died of AIDS only holds for a particular subset of homosexual men (i.e. those likely to acquire AIDS through a high number of frequently changing sexual partners with whom anal receptive sexual techniques were performed [51, 52]. This possibility that an enlarged SCN may be related to, for example, the level of sexual activity rather than to homosexuality warrants further study. However, experiments in rats have shown a close correlation between sexual activity and SDN size [11]. Our observation that the size of the SDN in homosexual men did not differ from that of the male reference group nor from that of the heterosexual men who died of AIDS does not support this possibility.

An alternative explanation for the enlarged SCN found in male homosexuals who had died of AIDS is that it might be related to the hypogonadism in adulthood that has been found in AIDS patients [53]. Our observation that the SCN in heterosexual male AIDS patients is not enlarged seems to exclude this possible explanation, but homosexual men who had not died of AIDS should certainly be studied in the future. In this respect, it is interesting that we observed an enlarged SCN in two (primary) male-to-female transsexuals who did not suffer from AIDS [36] (fig. 5).

The functional implications of the association between sexual orientation in men and SCN size are not clear. Various observations in animals suggest that the SCN, apart from being the biological clock, may be involved in reproductive processes [35, 36]. Judged from its nucleolar size, the SCN is also activated around puberty in rats [54]. In addition, lesions of the SCN area in the female rat attenuated the positive feedback response of gonadotrophic hormones to oestrogens [55, 56]. However, recently it was observed that lesions in the adult male rat SCN did not alter sexual orientation [F.H. De Jonge et al., unpubl. observ.]. This observation argues in favour of the possibility that sexual orientation and the size of the SCN are not causally related, but may be subject to the same organizing factor in development. The relationship between a large SCN and homosexuality is unexpected and difficult to interpret. The relationship need not be causal, in the sense that it is a necessary and sufficient condition for developing a homosexual orientation. It is imperative to study more material before definitive conclusions can be drawn. We have no information on the size of the SCN in female homosexuals or bisexuals. Until more data have been collected our finding is open to interpretation. It is particularly pertinent to study the SDN and SCN in subjects whose prenatal and postnatal history has been atypical (for example an excess of androgens in females or a deficiency or insensitivity to

Table 1. Results from the study of three transsexual subjects (T1, T2, T3)

	T1	T2	T3
Hypothalamus	Large SCN; small SDN	Large SCN; small SDN	Small SCN; large SDN
Male-to-female	Gender dysphoria from early childhood onwards	Gender dysphoria from early childhood onwards	Gender dysphoria postpubertally
Sexual/social orientation	Androphile, married under social pressure, father, last 4 years of life gynaephilic, hostile towards men	Asexual but surrounded herself with women	Gynaephilic, father following operation asexual
Hormone treatment	Cyproterone acetate, ethinylestradiol	Cyproterone acetate, stilbestrol ethinylestradiol	Cyproterone acetate, ethinylestradiol
Age at death (years)	50	44	43
Cause of death	Suicide	Probably cardiovascular	Sarcoma

androgens in males) as has been done in earlier work on sexual orientation (e.g. Money et al. [57]).

Transsexuality

It has been proposed that gender identity, like sexual orientation, develops as a result of an interaction between the developing brain and sex hormones. Transsexuality is considered to be the result of a disturbance of this interaction [6, 45]. In view of the similarity between the hypotheses on the development of gender and sexual orientation, it is of interest that 60% of male-to-female transsexuals are androphile and 10% are biphile. In 95% of cases, female-to-male transsexuals are gynaecophilic [58]. These data indicate that similar (but as yet unknown) mechanisms may play a role in the development of both gender and sexual orientation.

We were given the opportunity to study the hypothalami of three male-to-female transsexuals (fig. 5, table 1). Two of them (T1, T2) appeared to have a large SCN with high cell numbers and a small SDN with low cell numbers. The third transsexual subject (T3) revealed exactly the opposite (i.e. a small SCN and a large SDN). These two different patterns could not be related to the sexual orientation of these three subjects (table 1) in any simple way. Table 1 suggests that a relationship might exist between a large SCN and small SDN and primary transsexuality (i.e. awareness of the gender problems from early childhood onwards) on the one hand, and a small SCN and large SDN and secondary transsexuality (i.e. awareness of transsexuality later in life) on the other. It will be obvious that more data are necessary in order to establish whether such a relationship exists.

Conclusions and Summary

Following observations in many mammalian species, the human hypothalamus is believed to undergo sexual differentiation during development, due to an organizing effect of sex hormones.

We have found a SDN in the preoptic area of the human hypothalamus that contains about twice as many cells in young adult men as in women. The magnitude of the sex difference in the SDN depends on age. In the literature two other hypothalamic nuclei (INAH-2 and -3) and a part of the bed nucleus of the stria terminalis have been reported to be sexually dimorphic in humans.

At term, the SDN contains only 20% of the cell number found at 2–4 years of age. The cell number rapidly increases in boys and girls, at the same rate, until 2–4 years of age, after which the SDN differentiates according to sex, due to a decrease in cell numbers in girls. This period of sexual differentiation of the human hypothalamus is much later than generally presumed in the literature, and reveals the possibility of postnatal factors such as hormones, other chemical compounds and psychosocial factors interacting in the sexual differentiation of the brain. A few preliminary observations in clinical conditions with deficient hormonal production suggest that the size and cell number of the human SDN in adulthood is influenced by sex hormones during development.

No difference in SDN cell number was observed between homosexual and heterosexual men. This refutes Dörner's hypothesis that male homosexuals have a 'female hypothalamus'.

In a sample of brains of homosexual men we found that the SCN contained twice as many cells as in the reference group. The observation that a similarly enlarged SCN was present in a woman with Prader-Willi syndrome suggests that sex hormones and SCN development might be interrelated. A recent report claimed INAH-3 to be more than twice as large in heterosexual men as in homosexual men. Preliminary data suggest that the SCN is large and the SDN small in primary male-to-female transsexuals and that the SCN is small and the SDN large in secondary male-to-female transsexuals, but more data have to be collected to confirm this observation.

In conclusion, differences in size and cell number have been reported in a number of hypothalamic nuclei in relation to sexual orientation and gender. However, the functional implications of these findings are far from clear.

Acknowledgements

Brain material was obtained from the Netherlands Brain Bank (coordinator Dr R. Ravid) and from Dr L.J.G. Gooren (Department of Endocrinology, Free University, Amsterdam, The Netherlands), Dr R.S. Williams (Neuropathology Laboratory, Shriver Center, Walton, USA), Dr L. Mrzljak and Dr I. Kostovic (Department of Anatomy, University of Zagreb, Yugoslavia), Dr P.G. Barth (Department of Pediatrics and Neurology, AMC, University of Amsterdam, The Netherlands) and Dr H.P.H. Kremer (Department of Neurology, University of Leyden, The Netherlands). General pathology and neuropathology were performed either at the Free University of Amsterdam (Dr W. Kamphorst) or at the AMC, University of Amsterdam (Dr D. Troost). We thank B. Fisser for his technical assistance and W. Verweij for her secretarial help.

References

1 Reyes FI, Boroditsky RS, Winter JSD, et al: Studies on human sexual development. II. Fetal and maternal serum gonadotropin and sex steroid concentrations. J Clin Endocrinol Metab 1974;38:612–617.
2 Winter JSD: Prepubertal and pubertal endocrinology; in Falkner F, Tanner JM (eds): Human Growth. I. Principles and Prenatal Growth. London, Baillière Tindall, 1978, vol 2, pp 183–213.
3 Swaab DF, Hofman MA: Sexual differentiation of the human brain. A historical perspective; in De Vries GJ, De Bruin JPC, Uylings HBM, et al (eds): Sex Differences in the Brain. Progress in Brain Research. Amsterdam, Elsevier, 1984, vol 61, pp 361–374.
4 Dörner G: Psychoneuroendocrine aspects of brain development and reproduction; in Zichella L, Pancheri P (eds): Psychoneuroendocrinology in Reproduction, an Interdisciplinary Approach. Amsterdam, Elsevier, 1979, pp 43–54.
5 Dörner G: Hormone-dependent brain development and preventive medicine. Monogr Neural Sci 1986;12:17–27.
6 Gladue BA, Green R, Helleman RE: Neuroendocrine response to oestrogen and sexual orientation. Science 1984;225:1496–1499.
7 Dörner G, Staudt J: Vergleichende morphologische Untersuchungen der Hypothalamusdifferenzierung bei Ratte und Mensch. Endokrinologie 1972;59:152–155.
8 Nordeen EJ, Nordeen KW, Sengelaub PR, et al: Androgens prevent normally occurring cell death in a sexually dimorphic spinal nucleus. Science 1985;229:671–673.
9 Swaab DF, Hofman MA: Sexual differentiation of the human hypothalamus: Ontogeny of the sexually dimorphic nucleus of the preoptic area. Dev Brain Res 1988;44:314–318.
10 Gorski RA, Gordon JH, Shryne JE, et al: Evidence for a morphological sex difference within the medial preoptic area of the rat brain. Brain Res 1978;148:333–346.
11 Anderson RH, Fleming DE, Rhees RW, et al: Relationship between sexual activity, plasma testosterone and the volume of the sexually dimorphic nucleus of the preoptic area in prenatally stressed and non-stressed rats. Brain Res 1986;370:1–10.
12 Turkenburg JL, Swaab DF, Endert E, et al: Effects of lesions of the sexually dimorphic nucleus on sexual behaviour of testosterone-treated female Wistar rats. Brain Res Bull 1988;22:215–224.
13 De Jonge FH, Louwerse AL, Ooms MP, et al: Lesions of the SDN-POA inhibit sexual behaviour of male Wistar rats. Brain Res Bull 1989;23:483–492.
14 Swaab DF, Fliers E: A sexually dimorphic nucleus – the human brain. Science 1985;228:1112–1115.
15 Hofman MA, Swaab DF: The sexually dimorphic nucleus of the preoptic area in the human brain: A comparative morphometric study. J Anat 1989;164:55–72.
16 Braak H, Braak E: The hypothalamus of the human adult: Chiasmatic region. Anat Embryol 1987;176:315–330.
17 Brockhaus H: Beitrag zur normalen Anatomie des Hypothalamus und der Zona incerta bei Menschen. J Psychol Neurol 1942;51:96–196.
18 Feremutsch K: Strukturanalyse des menschlichen Hypothalamus. Monatsschr Psychiatr Neurol 1955;121:87–113.
19 Feremutsch K: Die Variabilität der cytoarchitektonischen Struktur des menschlichen Hypothalamus. Monatsschr Psychiatr Neurol 1948;116:257–283.
20 Allen LS, Hines M, Shryne JE, et al: Two sexually dimorphic cell groups in the human brain. J Neurosci 1989;9:497–506.
21 LeVay S: A difference in hypothalamic structure between heterosexual and homosexual men. Science 1991;253:1034–1037.
22 Allen LS, Gorski RA: Sex difference in the bed nucleus of the stria terminalis of the human brain. J Comp Neurol 1990;302:697–706.
23 Swaab DF, Fliers E, Partiman TS: The suprachiasmatic nucleus of the human brain in relation to sex, age and senile dementia. Brain Res 1985;342:37–44.
24 Polzovic A, Marinkovic R, Gudovic R, et al: Vascularizaton of the preoptic area in the human fetus; in Bajic M (ed): Advances in the Biosciences. Neuron, Brain and Behaviour. Oxford, Pergamon Press, 1988, vol 70, pp 143–146.
25 Abramovich DR, Davidson IA, Longstaff A, et al: Sexual differentiation of the human midtrimester brain. Eur J Obstet Gynecol Reprod Biol 1987;25:7–14.
26 Forest M, Cathiard AM: Patterns of plasma testosterone and 4-androstenedione in normal newborns: Evidence for testicular activity at birth. J Clin Endocrinol Metab 1975;41:977–981.
27 Gooren LJG, Fliers E, Courtney K: Biological determinants of sexual orientation. Ann Rev Sex Res 1990;1:175–196.
28 Gooren LJG, Cohen-Kettenis P: Erotosexuality in a man lacking physiological postnatal androgen exposure. J Psychol Hum Sexuality 1988;1:129–135.

29 Bray GA, Dahms WT, Swerdloff RS, et al: The Prader-Willi syndrome: A study of 40 patients and a review of the literature. Medicine 1983;62:59–80.
30 Knorr D, Weil J: Klinefelter's syndrome: Diagnostic criteria in childhood; in Bandmann H-J, Breit R (eds): Klinefelter's Syndrome. Berlin, Springer Verlag, 1984, pp 29–39.
31 Vogt H-J: Sexual behaviour in Klinefelter's syndrome; in Bandmann H-J, Breit R (eds): Klinefelter's Syndrome. Berlin, Springer Verlag 1984, pp 163–169.
32 Moore RY: Central neural control of circadian rhythms; in Ganong WF, Martini L (eds): Frontiers in Neuroendocrinology. New York, Raven Press, 1978, vol 5, pp 185–206.
33 Rusak B, Zucker I: Neural regulation of circadian rhythms. Physiol Rev 1979;59:449–526.
34 Moore-Ede MC, Sulzman FM, Fuller CA: The Clocks that Time Us. Physiology of the Circadian Timing System. Cambridge, MA, Harvard University Press, 1982.
35 Södersten P, Hansen S, Srebro B: Suprachiasmatic lesions disrupt the daily rhythmicity in the sexual behaviour of normal male rats and of male rats treated neonatally with antioestrogen. J Endocrinol 1981;88:125.
36 Swaab DF, Roozendaal B, Ravid R, et al: Suprachiasmatic nucleus in ageing, Alzheimer's disease, transsexuality and Prader-Willi syndrome; in de Kloet ER, Wiegant VM, De Wied D (eds): Neuropeptides and Brain Function. Progress in Brain Research. Amsterdam, Elsevier 1987, vol 72, pp 301–311.
37 Swaab DF, Hofman MA: An enlarged suprachiasmatic nucleus in homosexual men. Brain Res 1990;537:141–148.
38 Ehrhardt AA, Meyer-Bahlburg HFL, Rosen LR: Sexual orientation after prenatal exposure to exogenous oestrogen. Arch Sex Behav 1985; 14:57–75.
39 Dörner G, Geiser T, Ahrens L, et al: Prenatal stress and possible aetiogenetic factor homosexuality in human males. Endokrinologie 1980;75:365–368.
40 McCormick CM, Witelson SF, Kingstone E: Left-handedness in homosexual men and women: Neuroendocrine implications. Psychoneuroendocrinology 1990;15:69–76.
41 Ellis L, Ames MA, Peckham W, et al: Sexual orientation of human offspring may be altered by severe maternal stress during pregnancy. J Sex Res 1988;25:152–157.
42 Bailey JM, Willerman L, Parks C: A test of the maternal stress theory of human male homosexuality. Arch Soc Behav 1991;20:277–293.
43 Schmidt G, Clement U: Does peace prevent homosexuality? Arch Sex Behav 1990;19: 183–187.
44 Swaab DF, Mirmiran M: Functional teratogenic effects of chemicals on the developing brain; in Cohen MM (ed): Monographs in Neural Sciences. Basel, Karger, 1986, vol 12, pp 45–57.
45 Dörner G: Neuroendocrine response to estrogen and brain differentiation in heterosexuals, homosexuals, and transsexuals. Arch Sex Behav 1988;17:57–75.
46 Gooren LJG: The neuroendocrine response of luteinizing hormone to estrogen administration in heterosexual, homosexual and transsexual subjects. J Clin Endocrinol Metab 1986;63: 583–588.
47 Gooren LJG: The neuroendocrine response of luteinizing hormone to estrogen administration in the human is not sex specific but dependent on the hormonal environment. J Clin Endocrinol Metab 1986;63:589–593.
48 Gooren LJG: The endocrinology of transsexualism: A review and commentary. Psychoneuroendocrinology 1990;15:3–14.
49 Hofman MA, Fliers E, Goudsmit E, et al: Morphometric analysis of the suprachiasmatic and paraventricular nuclei in the human brain. J Anat 1988;160:127–143.
50 Swaab DF, Hofman MA, Honnebier MBOM: Development of vasopressin neurons in the human suprachiasmatic nucleus in relation to birth. Dev Brain Res 1990;52:289–293.
51 Curran JW, Meade Morgan W, Hardy AM, et al: The epidemiology of AIDS: Current status and future prospects. Science 1985;229: 1352–1357.
52 Van Griensven GJP, Tielman RAP, Goudsmit J, et al: Risk factors and prevalence of HIV antibodies in homosexual men in The Netherlands. Am J Epidemiol 1987;125:1048–1057.
53 Croxson TS, Chapman WE, Miller LK, et al: Changes in the hypothalamic-pituitary-gonadal axis in human immunodeficiency virus-infected homosexual men. J Clin Endocrinol Metab 1989;68:317–321.
54 Anderson CH: Nucleolus: Changes at puberty in neurons of the suprachiasmatic nucleus and the preoptic area. Exp Neurol 1981;74: 780–786.
55 Gray GD, Södersten P, Tallentrie D, et al: Effects of lesions in various structures of the suprachiasmatic-preoptic region on LH regulation and sexual behaviour in female rats. Neuroendocrinology 1978;25:174–191.
56 Wiegand SJ, Terasawa E, Bridson WE, et al: Effects of discrete lesions of preoptic and suprachiasmatic structures in the female rat: Alterations in the feedback regulation of gonadotropin secretion. Neuroendocrinology 1980;31:147–157.
57 Money J, Schwartz M, Lewis VG: Adult erotosexual status and fetal hormonal masculinization: 46,XX congenital virilizing adrenal hyperplasia and 46,XY androgen-insensitivity syndrome compared. Psychoneuroendocrinology 1984;9:405–414.
58 Coleman E, Bockting WO, Gooren LJG: Homosexual and bisexual identity in sex-reassigned female-to-male transsexuals. Arch Sex Behav 1992; in press.

Horm Res 1992;38(suppl 2):62–65

J.R. Hawkins

Imperial Cancer Research Fund,
London, UK

Genetic Determinants of Testis Development in Normal and Abnormal Individuals

Key Words
SRY
TDF
Testis determination
XX males
XY females

Abstract
A candidate for the male sex determining gene 2 has recently been isolated. This gene, named *SRY*, has an expression profile consistent with a role in testis determination, is mutated in some XY females, and causes female to male sex reversal in transgenic mice. The cloning of this gene should facilitate the characterization of other genes in the testis determining pathway.

Introduction

There are two main themes in mammalian sex determination. The first is the role of the Y chromosome and the second is the role of the testis. It has long been known that females have two X chromosomes and males have an X and a Y. Insight into how these 'sex' chromosomes relate to gender was provided by the study of individuals with abnormal sex chromosome constitutions. In the absence of the Y chromosome, individuals with one, two, three, or four X chromosomes are female; individuals with one or more Y chromosomes, irrespective of the number of X chromosomes, are male [1, 2]. Thus, the Y chromosome acts as a dominant inducer of maleness. Knowledge of the central role of the testis in sex determination stems from a series of surgical experiments conducted by Jost in the 1940s [3]. When Jost removed the developing testes from young rabbit embryos, he found that these rabbits developed as females. Similarly, when the developing ovaries of female rabbit embryos were removed, those rabbits also developed as females. These observations imply that it is the presence or absence of testes that dictates the sex of a mammal, and that male sexual characteristics are under hormonal control of the testes. It appears, therefore, that a gene or genes on the Y chromosome is responsible for the testis and hence male development. This genetic entity has been named the testis determining factor (*TDF*) in humans and testis determining Y gene (*Tdy*) in mice. It should be stressed that *TDF/Tdy* is not solely responsible for testicular development but is one of many genes involved in a complex genetic pathway. The only way in which *TDF/Tdy* differs from the other genes involved is in its location on the Y chromosome.

A Strategy for Cloning *TDF*

Attempts to clone *TDF* have relied on positional information of the gene, derived from XX males. In male meiosis the X and Y chromosomes pair at the tips of their short arms in a region known as the pseudoautosomal region (PAR), and this pairing is essential for correct segregation of the X and Y chromosomes. In every male meiotic event a single recombination occurs in the PAR. In rare instances, however, the recombination event extends beyond the pseudoautosomal region, transferring X- and Y-specific DNA between the sex chromosomes. Such aberrant recombinations, extending beyond *TDF*, result in X

J.R. Hawkins
Imperial Cancer Research Fund
44 Lincoln's Inn Fields
London WC2A 3PX (UK)

0301–0163/92/0388–0062
$ 2.75/0

chromosomes carrying *TDF* (producing XX males) and Y chromosomes that have lost *TDF* (producing XY females). Different XX males are seen to carry differing amounts of Y-DNA (fig. 1). *TDF* must be present in all Y-DNA positive XX males and must, therefore, reside in the region immediately centromeric to the pseudoautosomal boundary (fig. 1). This 35 kb region was cloned and searched for genes; only one candidate sequence was identified. This sequence when used as a probe on 'Noah's Ark blots' revealed a Y-linked homologue in all eutherian mammals tested (fig. 2) [4]. The DNA sequence of this fragment revealed a 669-base pair open reading frame, with the potential to encode a 79-amino acid high mobility group (HMG) box domain – a known DNA binding motif. This gene, named sex determining region Y gene (*SRY*) was therefore proposed as a candidate for *TDF*.

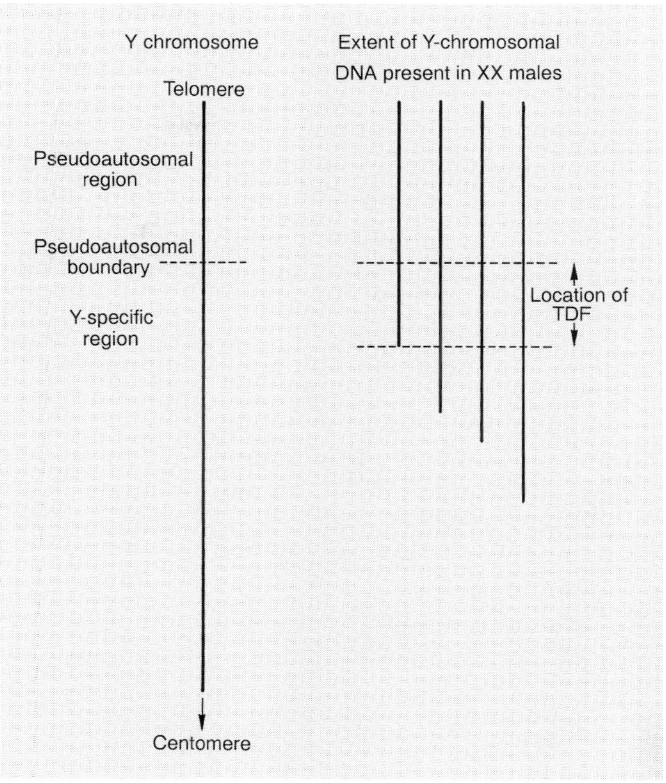

Fig. 1. A schematic diagram showing the variable size of Y-chromosomal fragments present in Y-DNA positive XX males. *TDF* resides in the region present in all these patients, immediately centromeric to the pseudoautosomal boundary.

SRY – A Candidate for *TDF*

For reasons of ethics and experimental simplicity, embryonic expression studies of *SRY* have been performed on its murine homologue, *Sry*. The *Sry* gene in the embryonic mouse is expressed exclusively in the genital ridge. Expression is first detectable at 10.5 days post coitum (dpc), peaks at 11.5 dpc, and is turned off after 12.5 dpc. This expression profile of *Sry* is consistent with a role in testis determination, as expression immediately precedes the first visible signs of testis differentiation, which occurs at 12.5 dpc. By studying *Sry* expression in W^e/W^e (germ cell deficient) mice, it has been determined that embryonic *Sry* transcripts are derived from the somatic portion of the gonad and not the germ cells, which are known to have no influence on sex determination [5].

Equivalence between *SRY/Sry* and *TDF/Tdy*

It was clear at this point that *SRY* was a good candidate for the testis determining gene, *TDF*, so efforts were directed at proving this hypothesis. Proof should come in the form of answers to two questions: (1) Is *SRY/Sry* required for testis determination?, and (2) is *SRY/Sry* sufficient to direct testis determination?

Mutational Analysis of XY Females

The first question could be answered by disrupting the *Sry* gene in mice or by looking for mutations in human patients with failed testis development (i.e. XY females). Certain XY females are the result of Y chromosome deletions caused by abnormal X-Y exchange. Most appear, however, to have intact Y chromosomes and could have resulted from point mutations in *TDF*. We searched for mutations in *SRY* in the genomes of XY females using the single strand conformational polymorphism (SSCP) assay. This is a simple procedure (based on the polymerase chain reaction) that is capable of detecting point mutations. Of 11 XY females tested, two gave abnormal SSCP patterns (fig. 3) [6]. The father of one, AA, had a normal pattern and the father of the other, JN, shared the abnormal pattern. The *SRY* genes of these two XY females and their fathers were sequenced. AA was seen to have a G to A base change causing a methionine to isoleucine amino acid substitution. This mutation, as predicted from the SSCP data, was not present in the father, implying that a de novo mutation had occurred and, by correlation of phenotype and genotype, that *SRY* is required for testis development. Less expected was the fact that the JN mutation – a G to C base change causing a valine to leucine amino acid substitu-

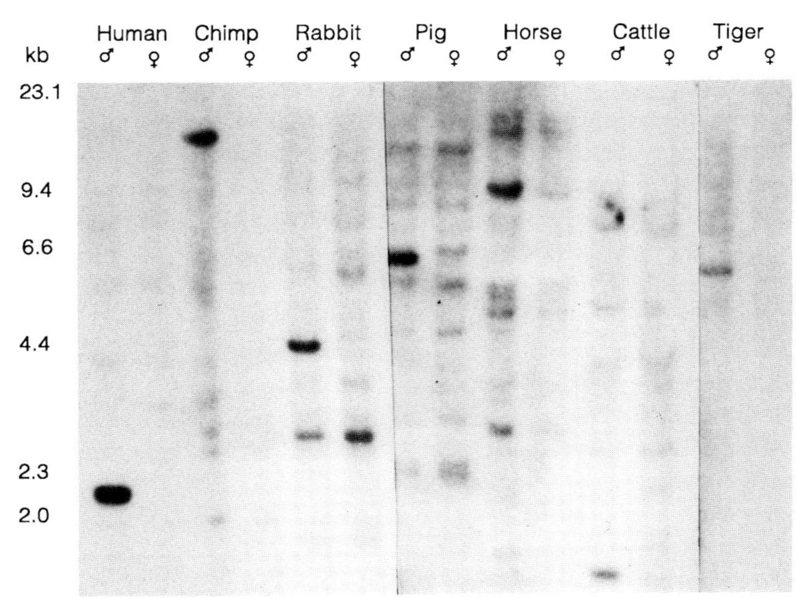

Fig. 2. 'Noah's Ark' Southern blot of HindIII digested genomic DNA from male and female pairs of eutherian mammals, hybridized with *SRY*. The probe detects male-specific fragments in each species. The rabbit female lane is slightly overloaded. Reproduced with permission from [4].

tion – was shared by her father. There were three possible explanations: (1) The alteration could be low frequency polymorphism and unrelated to the phenotype; (2) the alteration is sex reversing and the father mosaic; (3) the alteration is conditionally sex reversing. Further analysis of this family revealed the father to have an XY female sister [7]. Therefore, the second explanation cannot be correct. Data described later will address explanations (1) and (3).

Recently the *SRY* gene from an additional 23 XY females has been sequenced by our group and a further 5 mutations identified. All of these mutations lie in the HMG box. Those XY females not mutant for *SRY* can be explained by mutations in other genes in the testis determining pathway.

The potential DNA-binding capacity of *SRY* has been studied in gel retardation experiments. Recombinant *SRY* protein was produced from 5 known *SRY* mutant XY females. Three of these 5 mutations are de novo, and 2 (1 of which is JN) are inherited. The normal *SRY* protein produced a 'band-shift' [8] with a specific heptamer DNA sequence in oligo probes known to be the target of TCF-1, another protein with an HMG box. This DNA-binding capacity was seen to be lost in four out of the 5 mutants and drastically reduced in the 5th. One of the 4 mutants to have its *SRY* DNA-binding capacity abolished was mutant JN. This indicates that the gene alteration in this individual is not a polymorphism, but indeed a mutation that is conditionally sex reversing. The mutant to have a reduced DNA-binding capacity is the other inherited mutant. Thus, in this case, there is a ready explanation for the incomplete penetrance of this mutation. In reality,

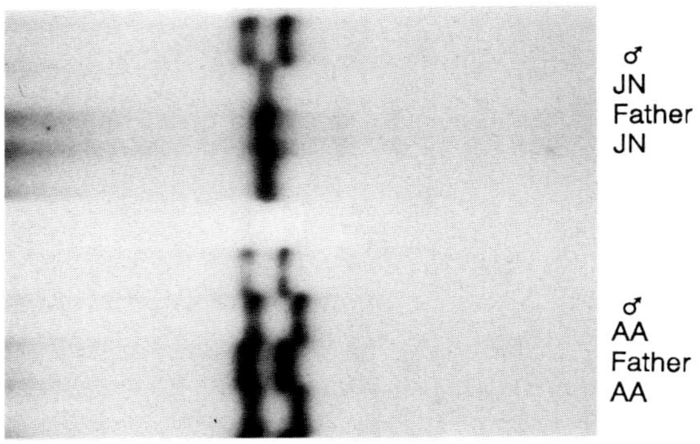

Fig. 3. Single strand conformational polymorphism analysis of *SRY* in XY females. In the upper portion is family N with control male; DNA from the father is flanked on each side by DNA of his XY daughter (JN). In the lower portion is family A with control male; again DNA from the father is flanked by that of his XY daughter (AA). (AA) and (JN) both have pure gonadal dysgenesis. Fifty normal males were tested as controls and no variation was detected. Reproduced with permission from [6].

mutant JN may also have some *SRY* activity, but is not demonstrable by this crude technique. Taken together these results imply that the DNA-binding activity of *SRY* is required for its function in sex determination.

Many genetic diseases show variable penetrance within families, the cause of this being the pleiotropic effects of other genes. In the case of testis determination, there is no opportunity for a spectrum of phenotypes for a given mutation, only a male or female phenotype. Therefore, with the inherited mutations, gender is probably a chance affair, depending on both the number of *SRY* molecules in the right place at the right time and the activity of those molecules.

Transgenic Mice

The second question asked in attempting to equate *SRY/Sry* with *TDF/Tdy* was 'is *SRY/Sry* sufficient to direct testis determination?' This question addresses whether *SRY/Sry* is the only gene required for testis determination on the Y chromosome. It was answered by producing mice transgenic for *Sry*. Some of the XX (chromosomally female) mice transgenic for *Sry* developed as males, formally proving that *Sry* is the only component of the Y chromosome required for testis determination [9].

It is, therefore, apparent that *SRY/Sry* is indeed *TDF/Tdy*. By cloning *SRY/Sry*, we now have a key for entering the testis determining pathway. Our understanding of the molecular events in mammalian sex determination is just beginning.

Acknowledgements

This work is the result of experiments performed over several years by many individuals in the laboratories of Peter Goodfellow and Robin Lovell-Badge. Much of its success has been due to the marriage of human genetics with mouse developmental biology in the form of a close collaboration between these two laboratories.

References

1 Ford CE, Jones KW, Polani P, et al: A sex chromosome anomaly in a case of gonadal sex dysgenesis (Turner's syndrome). Lancet 1959; i:711–713.

2 Jacobs FA, Strong JA: A case of human intersexuality having a possible XXY sex determining mechanism. Nature 1959;183:320–303.

3 Jost A, Vigier B, Prepin J, et al: Studies on sex differentiation in mammals. Recent Prog Horm Res 1973;29:1–14.

4 Sinclair AH, Berta P, Palmer MS, et al: A gene from the human sex-determining region encodes a protein with homology to a conserved DNA-binding motif. Nature 1990;346: 240–244.

5 Koopman P, Munserberg A, Capel B, et al: Expression of a candidate sex-determining gene during mouse testis differentiation. Nature 1990;348:450–452.

6 Berta P, Hawkins JR, Sinclair AH, et al: Genetic evidence equating *SRY* and the testis determining factor. Nature 1990;348:448–450.

7 McElreavey K, Vilain N, Abbas N, et al: XY females with conditional mutation of SRY in the testis-determining regions suggests other sex-determining genes in humans. Cytogenet Cell Genet 1991;58:2093.

8 Harley VR, Jackson DI, Hextall PJ, et al: Sequence-specific DNA binding by the human sex determining gene product, *SRY*, is abolished by mutation in some XY females. Science (in press).

9 Koopman R, Gubbay J, Vivian N, et al: Male development of chromosomally female mice transgenic for *Sry*. Nature 1991;351:117–121.

Horm Res 1992;38(suppl 2):66–71

R. Voutilainen

Departments of Pediatrics and Pathology,
University of Helsinki, Finland

Differentiation of the Fetal Gonad

Key Words
Anti-Müllerian hormone
Gonadotrophins
Inhibins
Ovary
Steroidogenesis
Testis

Abstract
Gonadal differentiation may be divided into four stages: pregonadal, indifferent, primary sex differentiation, and secondary sex differentiation. Sertoli cells appear at 6–7 weeks and Leydig cells differentiate at 8 weeks, but in ovaries, primary sex differentiation occurs much later. Testosterone secretion peaks at 12–16 weeks causing male secondary sex development together with the appearance of anti-Müllerian hormone. Fetal testis is able to synthesize and secrete inhibins. Lower circulating luteinizing hormone (LH) and follicle stimulating hormone (FSH) levels in male than in female fetuses at midgestation suggest that the fetal pituitary is already responsive to the gonadal hormones. Placental human chorionic gonadotrophin may regulate testosterone synthesis at midgestation, and both LH and FSH are likely to have some regulatory effect on fetal gonads during the last third of gestation.

Introduction

Sex is determined genetically at conception. The presence of the testis determining factor guides gonadal differentiation to the formation of testes. Two testicular hormones, anti-Müllerian hormone (AMH) and testosterone, are needed for normal development of male internal and external genitalia. The differentiation of the indifferent gonad to the ovary, or the absence of gonads, leads to the female type differentiation. Thus, female sexual development is spontaneous and ovarian hormonal activity is not needed for normal female development during fetal life.

Morphological Development of the Gonad

Morphological sexual development may be divided into four stages: the pregonadal stage, the indifferent stage, primary sexual differentiation and secondary sexual differentiation [1, 2]. The pregonadal stage begins with differentiation of primordial germ cells in the 4.5-day-old blastocyst. No gonadal structures exist at this stage, but the ultimate development of female or male gonads has already been predetermined by the chromosomal sex or, more accurately, by the presence or absence of the testis determining factor.

The period of the indifferent gonad begins with the development of the gonadal ridges and lasts about 7–10 days. The indifferent gonad begins as a stage of rapid proliferation and thickening of the genital ridge and its coelomic epithelium. At the same time the primordial germ cells start to migrate from the yolk sac to the coelomic epithelium of the urogenital ridge. By 5–6 weeks of gestation, the indifferent gonad is composed of primordial germ cells, supporting cells of the coelomic epithelium, and the mesenchyme of the gonadal ridge.

One of the first morphological signs of male primary sex differentiation is the appearance of Sertoli cells at 6–7 weeks. Testicular cords are formed by aggregation of Sertoli cells and the germ cells are later enclosed within the cords. Germ cells not enclosed by testicular cords rapidly degenerate. The differentiation of mesenchymal somatic

R. Voutilainen
Department of Pediatrics
University of Helsinki, Children's Hospital
Stenbäckinkatu 11
SF–00290 Helsinki (Finland)

0301–0163/92/0388–0066
$ 2.75/0

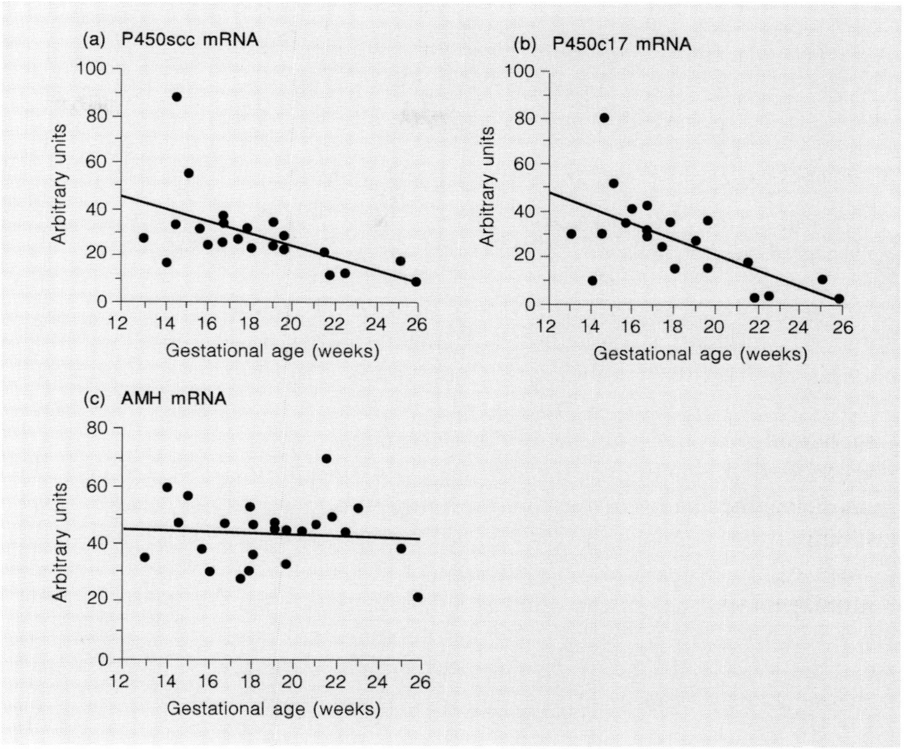

Fig. 1. Developmental pattern of (**a**) P450scc, (**b**) P450c17 and (**c**) anti-Müllerian hormone (AMH) gene expression in human fetal testes. Linear regression analysis shows that P450scc and c17 mRNAs decrease significantly during the second trimester, but AMH mRNA remains unchanged. (Modified from references 4 and 5.)

cells into Leydig cells follows at 8 weeks. The lack of differentiation of Sertoli cells can be regarded as a sign of ovarian development. Active ovarian development from the indifferent gonad occurs much later than the development of testicular cords in the male gonad.

During secondary sex differentiation, the endocrine and paracrine effects of testicular hormones (testosterone from the Leydig cells and AMH from the Sertoli cells) cause the stabilization of the Wolffian structures and the regression of the Müllerian ducts in the male fetus. In the absence of the testicular hormones, the Müllerian ducts remain and female-type internal and external genitalia develop. In the testes, Sertoli cells surrounding the germ cells make up the majority of the testicular cord cells. Degenerating germ cells are removed by Sertoli cells. Only mitotic division of male germ cells occurs during fetal life: meiotic division is supposed to be inhibited by certain Sertoli cell product(s) (possibly AMH or inhibins). The number of Leydig cells at 14 weeks decreases substantially by birth.

In the female gonad, primitive germ cells are scattered throughout the ovarian parenchyma at 7–9 weeks of gestation. At 12 weeks, the ovarian cortex begins to thicken due to increased mitotic activity of the oogonia and the primitive granulosa cells. Primordial follicles (small oocytes surrounded by a single layer of flat granulosa cells and a basal membrane) can be seen from 13.5 weeks onwards. When granulosa cells become cuboidal and start to divide, primary follicles can be seen. Pre-antral follicles (enlarged oocytes each with a zona pellucida, multiple layers of granulosa cells and a thecal cell layer) can be seen from the sixth month onwards. Antral follicles (fully developed oocytes with a fluid-filled cavity and multiple layers of granulosa cells) may be seen near term and represent 0.1–0.5% of all follicles. The peak number of germ cells is reached at 16–20 weeks, with a progressive reduction thereafter. Oocytes of the same developmental stage can typically be seen for a long period of time. On the other hand, oocytes of different maturational stages are seen simultaneously. The mechanisms governing the individual maturational pace of oocytes is not known.

Hormonal Development of the Gonad

Steroid Hormone Synthesis in Fetal Testes

The onset of testosterone synthesis follows closely the histological differentiation of the Leydig cells at about 8 weeks of gestation. The testosterone content of fetal testes is highest at 12–14 weeks of gestation, with a clear decrease thereafter [3]. As the human chorionic gonadotrophin (hCG) concentration peaks in maternal and fetal circulation at about 10 weeks of gestation, and hCG receptors are present in fetal testes, it has been proposed that hCG is the physiological regulator of fetal testicular testosterone synthesis and secretion. The developmental pattern of testicular expression of two key steroidogenic enzyme genes, P450scc (cholesterol side-chain cleavage enzyme) and P450c17 (17-hydroxylase/17,20-lyase), follows the same pattern as testosterone concentration in fetal circulation and the number of hCG binding sites in fetal testes (fig. 1).

Steroid Hormone Synthesis in Fetal Ovaries

Fetal ovaries do not produce significant amounts of steroids during the first two trimesters. Although some aromatase activity has been detected in first and second trimester ovaries [6], the physiological significance of this is unclear, because the activities of the other steroidogenic enzymes are very low. The expression of all steroidogenic enzyme genes in second trimester human ovaries is very low: P450scc, P450c17 (fig. 2) [7], aromatase [8] and 3βHSD (3β-hydroxysteroid dehydrogenase) mRNAs (fig. 3) are all undetectable or at a very low level. The fetal ovary also lacks hCG [10] and follicle stimulating hormone (FSH) receptors [11] during the first two trimesters, again emphasizing the hormonal silence of the female gonad compared with its male counterpart.

AMH in Fetal Gonads

AMH is a testicular glycoprotein responsible for the regression of Müllerian ducts in the male fetus. This hormone is also called Müllerian inhibiting substance (MIS) or factor (MIF). It is produced by fetal testicular Sertoli cells. Müllerian ducts are responsive to the regressive effect of AMH only at a certain critical period of gestation. The AMH receptors have not, however, been characterized or cloned. Testicular production of AMH is maximal during the period of Müllerian duct regression in males, though it can be clearly detected throughout the remainder of gestation, and even during postnatal life [12]. The physiological functions, if any, that AMH may have after the period of Müllerian duct regression are not known. It has been suggested that it might function as an inhibitor of germ cell meiosis [13].

A pronounced expression of the AMH gene was found in human fetal testes, and no decrease of AMH mRNA was seen from 13 to 25 weeks of gestation (fig. 1), proving that the AMH gene remains switched on after the period of Müllerian duct regression. Fetal ovaries seemed to express

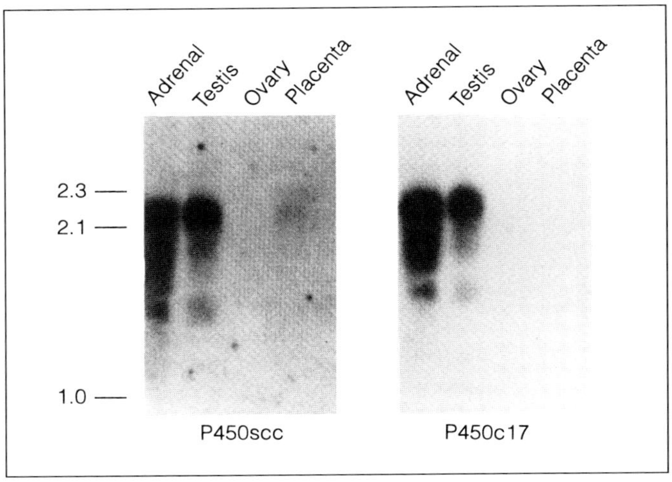

Fig. 2. Tissue-specific expression of P450scc and c17 genes in human fetal tissues. Northern blot of fetal RNA samples probed sequentially with labelled human cDNAs for P450scc and P450c17. Each lane contains 25 μg total RNA. Molecular weight markers are shown on the left. (Modified from reference 5.)

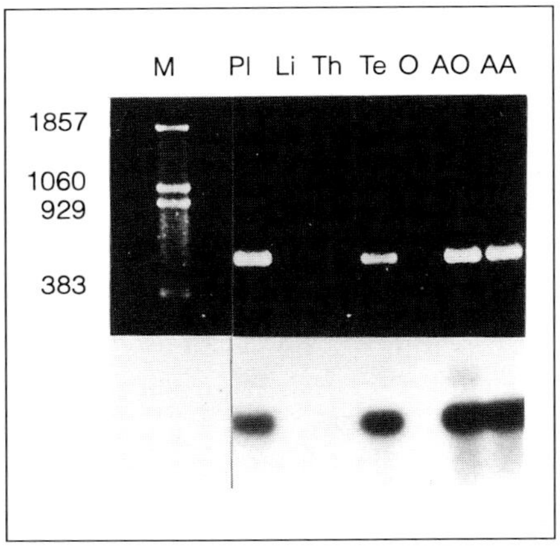

Fig. 3. Expression of 3β-hydroxysteroid dehydrogenase (3βHSD) gene in different tissues as analyzed by RT-PCR techniques. RNA (1 μg total) from each tissue was reverse transcribed to cDNA and then amplified using primers specific for human 3βHSD cDNA. Ethidium bromide stained agarose gel analysis after two 25 cycle rounds of amplification is shown in the upper part of the figure. The Southern blot of the gel was probed with an independent 3βHSD-specific ^{32}P-labelled probe; the autoradiograph is shown in the lower part of the figure. The RNA sources for RT-PCR reactions are shown at the top: Pl = placenta; Li = fetal liver; Th = fetal thyroid; Te = fetal testis; O = fetal ovary; AO = adult ovarian granulosa cells; AA = adult adrenal. (Modified from reference 9.)

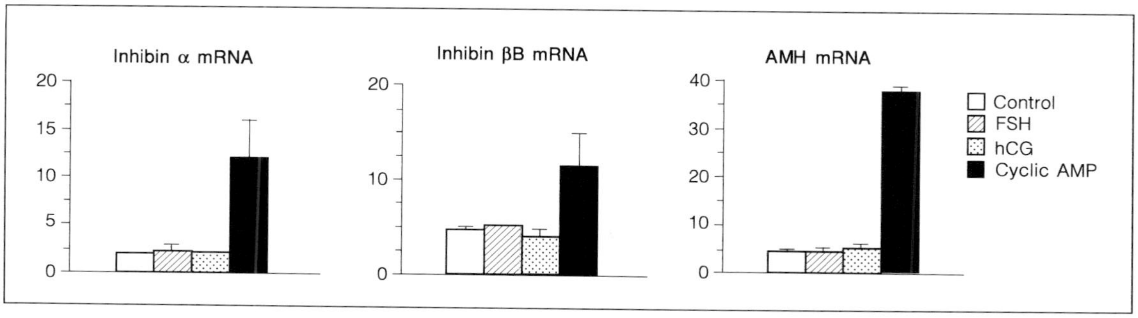

Fig. 4. Regulation of inhibin subunit and AMH mRNAs in primary cultures of human fetal testicular cells. Dispersed testicular cells were cultured for 5 days without any stimuli and then for 2 days with FSH (50 ng/ml), hCG (50 ng/ml) or dibutyryl cyclic AMP (0.2 m*M*). Triplicate wells were used for each stimulus, and means ± SEM of the scanning values from the dot blot autoradiograph are presented. The AMH data are modified from reference 4.

very little AMH mRNA (less than 2% of the testicular amount), based on dot blot analysis. However, more specific and sensitive techniques will be needed to verify this finding. It was interesting to see that human adult ovarian granulosa cells clearly expressed AMH mRNA and that this expression was up-regulated by gonadotrophins [4]. In cultured human fetal testicular cells, dibutyryl cyclic AMP treatment clearly induced AMH mRNA accumulation, but in our culture conditions at least FSH and hCG had no effect (fig.4).

Inhibins in Fetal Gonads

Inhibins are classically known as gonadal glycoprotein hormones inhibiting pituitary FSH secretion [14]. They are composed of an α-subunit and one of two β-subunits (βA or βB), joined by disulphide bonds. Both inhibins A (αβA) and B (αβB) preferentially inhibit FSH release from the pituitary, though dimers of the β-subunits (so-called activins) increase pituitary FSH secretion. Activin A is a homodimer of βA-subunits (βAβA), while activin B is a homodimer of βB-subunits (βBβB), and activin AB is a heterodimer of β-subunits (βAβB). Each of the inhibin/activin subunits is encoded by separate genes, and the primary translation products are further processed before they join to form mature inhibins or activins. Very little is known about the posttranscriptional regulation of inhibin/activin formation.

Inhibin subunit gene expression was detectable in fetal testes, adrenals and placenta [15–17], whereas fetal ovaries did not express any of the inhibin subunit genes during the second trimester. In testicular samples, α-subunit mRNA tended to decrease from 13 to 25 weeks of gestation. At the same time, βB-subunit mRNA remained at the same level. βA mRNA was not detectable by Northern or dot blot analysis in fetal testes.

In primary cultures of second trimester human fetal testicular cells, dibutyryl cyclic AMP treatment increased α mRNA about six-fold and βB mRNA 2.5-fold (fig.4) [15]. In testicular cultures, some βA mRNA could be detected in Northern and dot blots. In contrast to α and βB mRNA, βA mRNA seemed to decrease in response to dibutyryl cyclic AMP treatment. In our experimental conditions, FSH and hCG had no effect on inhibin subunit mRNAs. The regulation of inhibin subunit mRNAs was similar to AMH mRNA in cultured testicular cells (fig.4).

Aspects of the Regulation of Fetal Gonadal Hormonogenesis

It is evident that human fetal testis is hormonally very active from about 6–8 weeks of gestation, when the Sertoli and Leydig cells differentiate. This hormonal activity is highest during the first two trimesters, and clearly wanes towards the end of gestation. On the other hand, human fetal ovary differentiates much later, the first signs of morphological differentiation being seen at about 12–13 weeks. The hormonal activity of the fetal ovary is weak throughout gestation.

LH/hCG receptors (high affinity binding sites) have been demonstrated in human fetal testes from 10 to 11 weeks of gestation onwards. The hCG binding capacity of fetal testes is highest between 15 and 20 weeks [10]. Although certain studies have revealed that hCG can induce testosterone synthesis either in organ cultures [18] or fetal testicular homogenates [19, 20], several groups have been unable to demonstrate induction of testosterone secretion or steroidogenic gene expression by hCG in second trimester human fetal testicular homogenates or in cultured testicular cells [7, 21]. It is not yet known at what gestational age fully functional hCG receptors appear in fetal Leydig cells; the presence of specific hCG binding sites does not necessarily mean that hCG binding leads to the intracellular cyclic AMP-mediated signalling needed for induction of testosterone secretion. Thus, it is quite likely that the initiation of testosterone secretion from human fetal testes is independent of gonadotrophin control.

It seems that the testosterone-LH negative feedback is already functional during the second trimester. This view is supported by the finding that pituitary and serum LH concentrations are lower in male than in female fetuses during the second trimester [22, 23]. This sex difference disappears during the third trimester, when circulating testosterone concentrations are at the same level in both sexes [23].

Both AMH and inhibins are produced by Sertoli cells in the testes. Cyclic AMP-mediated mechanisms clearly increase both AMH and inhibin subunit gene expression in cultured human fetal testicular cells (fig. 4). FSH is the physiological regulator of Sertoli cells. In our experimental conditions at least, FSH was not able to increase AMH or inhibin subunit mRNAs. Although specific FSH binding sites have been demonstrated in human fetal testes from 9 to 11 weeks onwards, no cyclic AMP generation was detected in response to FSH binding [11]. This raises the possibility that the FSH receptors are not yet fully functional at this stage of development. Another possibility for the unresponsiveness of AMH and inhibin subunit mRNAs to gonadotrophins in these experiments could have been the loss of gonadotrophin receptors in cell culture conditions. As both AMH and inhibin genes are clearly expressed and these hormones are already secreted from fetal testes during the first trimester, there must be factors other than FSH controlling AMH and inhibin secretion during early differentiation of fetal testis. The fetal pituitary seems to be responsive to the negative effect of inhibin as pituitary and circulating FSH concentrations are clearly lower in male than in female fetuses during the second trimester [22, 23]. This sex difference disappears by the end of gestation, when the hormonal activity of the fetal testis decreases.

Although pituitary gonadotrophins are not important for the regulation of fetal gonadal function during the first two trimesters, they probably have some role in the maintenance of normal testicular and ovarian structure during the third trimester. This view is supported by the findings in anencephalic fetuses, who have normal gonadal development during the first half of gestation. In male anencephalic fetuses, a reduction in the number of Leydig cells has been detected with advancing gestation. In female anencephalic fetuses, the ovaries develop normally until week 32 of pregnancy. After that, a lack of antral follicles and a reduction in ovarian size has been detected (see [2] for references).

References

1 Wartenberg H: Differentiation and development of the testis; in Burger H, de Kretser D (eds): The Testis, Second Edition, New York, Raven Press, 1989, pp 67–118.

2 Rabinovici J, Jaffe RB: Development and regulation of growth and differentiated function in human and subhuman primate fetal gonads. Endocr Rev 1990;11:532–557.

3 Reyes FI, Winter JSD, Faiman C: Studies on human sexual development: I. Fetal gonadal and adrenal sex steroids. J Clin Endocrinol Metab 1973;37:74–78.

4 Voutilainen R, Miller WL: Human Müllerian inhibitory factor messenger ribonucleic acid is hormonally regulated in the fetal testis and in adult granulosa cells. Mol Endocrinol 1987;1: 604–608.

5 Voutilainen R, Miller WL: Developmental expression of genes for the steroidogenic enzymes P450scc (20,22 desmolase), P450c17 (17α-hydroxylase/17,20 lyase), and P450c21 (21-hydroxylase) in the human fetus. J Clin Endocrinol Metab 1986;63:1145–1150.

6 George FW, Wilson JD: Conversion of androgen to estrogen by the human fetal ovary. J Clin Endocrinol Metab 1978;47:550–555.

7 Voutilainen R, Miller WL: Developmental and hormonal regulation of mRNAs for insulin-like growth factor II and steroidogenic enzymes in human fetal adrenals and gonads. DNA 1988; 7:9–15.

8 Tapanainen J, Voutilainen R, Jaffe RB: Low aromatase activity and gene expression in human fetal testes. J Steroid Biochem 1989; 33:7–11.

9 Voutilainen R, Ilvesmäki V, Miettinen PJ: Low expression of 3β-hydroxy-5-ene steroid dehydrogenase gene in human fetal adrenals in vivo: Adrenocorticotrophin and protein kinase C dependent regulation in adrenocortical cultures. J Clin Endocrinol Metab 1991;72: 761–767.

10 Molsberry RL, Carr BR, Mendelson CR, et al: Human chorionic gonadotropin binding to human fetal testes as a function of gestational age. J Clin Endocrinol Metab 1982;55: 791–794.

11 Huhtaniemi IT, Yamamoto M, Ranta T, et al: Follicle-stimulating hormone receptors appear earlier in the primate fetal testis than in the ovary. J Clin Endocrinol Metab 1987;65: 1210–1214.

12 Tran D, Picard JY, Campargue J, et al: Immunocytochemical detection of anti-Müllerian hormone in Sertoli cells of various mammalian species including human. J Histochem Cytochem 1987;35:733–743.

13 Tran D, Picard JY, Vigier B, et al: Persistence of Müllerian ducts in male rabbits passively immunized against bovine anti-Müllerian hormone during fetal life. Dev Biol 1986;116: 160–167.

14 Ying S-Y: Inhibins, activins, and follistatins: Gonadal proteins modulating the secretion of follicle-stimulating hormone. Endocr Rev 1988;9:267–293.
15 Voutilainen R, Erämaa M: Hormonally regulated inhibin gene expression in human fetal adrenals and testes. Horm Res 1989;suppl 1:15 (Abstr 57).
16 Voutilainen R: Developmental aspects on hormonal regulation of Müllerian inhibitory factor and inhibins; in Westermark B, Betsholtz C, Hökfelt B (eds): Growth Factors in Health and Disease. Amsterdam, Elsevier Science Publishers, 1990, pp 43–52.
17 Voutilainen R, Erämaa M, Ritvos O: Hormonally regulated inhibin gene expression in human fetal and adult adrenals. J Clin Endocrinol Metab 1991;73:1026–1030.
18 Abramovich DR, Baker T, Neal P: Effect of human chorionic gonadotrophin on testosterone secretion by the foetal human testis in organ culture. J Endocrinol 1974;60:179–185.
19 Ahluwalia B, Williams J, Verma P: In vitro testosterone biosynthesis in the human fetal testis. II. Stimulation by cyclic AMP and human chorionic gonadotrophin (hCG). Endocrinology 1974;95:1411–1415.
20 Huhtaniemi IT, Korenbrot CC, Jaffe RB: hCG binding and stimulation of testosterone biosynthesis in the human fetal testis. J Clin Endocrinol Metab 1977;44:963–967.
21 Word RA, George FW, Wilson JD, et al: Testosterone synthesis and adenylate cyclase activity in the early human fetal testis appears to be independent of human chorionic gonadotrophin control. J Clin Endocrinol Metab 1989; 69:204–208.
22 Clements JA, Reyes FI, Winter JSD, Fairman C: Studies on human sexual development. III. Fetal pituitary and serum, and amniotic fluid concentrations of LH, CG, and FSH. J Clin Endocrinol Metab 1976;42:9–19.
23 Beck-Peccoz P, Padmanabhan V, Baggiani AM, et al: Maturation of hypothalamic-pituitary-gonadal function in normal human fetuses: Circulating levels of gonadotrophins, their common α-subunit and free testosterone, and discrepancy between immunological and biological activities of circulating follicle-stimulating hormone. J Clin Endocrinol Metab 1991;73:525–532.

Horm Res 1992;38(suppl 2):72–76

N. Josso

Unité de Recherches sur l'Endocrinologie
du Développement (INSERM)
Montrouge, France

Anti-Müllerian Hormone and Sertoli Cell Function

Key Words
Müllerian inhibiting substance
Müllerian inhibiting factor
Sertoli cells
Intersex states
Anorchia
Persistent Müllerian duct syndrome

Abstract
Anti-Müllerian hormone (AMH) is a glycoprotein that is produced by immature Sertoli cells and is responsible for the regression of Müllerian ducts in male fetuses. It is a useful marker of testicular function in children, when anorchia is suspected and in intersex states. In the persistent Müllerian duct syndrome, both AMH-positive and AMH-negative forms have been reported. In three cases of the latter, a mutation of the AMH gene is thought to have been responsible for the condition.

Introduction

Anti-Müllerian hormone (AMH), also called Müllerian inhibiting substance or Müllerian inhibiting factor, is a glycoprotein dimer member of the transforming growth factor-B family. It is synthesized by immature Sertoli cells and postnatal granulosa cells [1]. AMH plays a key role in male sex differentiation by inhibiting the development of female sex organs during fetal life. Although it continues to be produced by the testis until puberty, it has not been proved that AMH is of physiological importance during childhood. However, assaying during this period provides information concerning the functional value of Sertoli cells [2, 3].

AMH in Normal Children

An enzyme linked immunosorbent assay (ELISA) for the measurement of AMH in human serum has recently been developed by several groups, including our own [2], using recombinant human AMH generated at Biogen Inc. (Cambridge, MA). The pattern of AMH secretion in normal boys is shown in figure 1; no serum AMH is detectable in girls. AMH serum levels are high during the first 2 years of life, and slowly decrease until puberty, when AMH becomes undetectable. During puberty, serum AMH levels are correlated with the stage of pubertal maturation (fig. 2).

Serum AMH levels reflect the number and functional value of Sertoli cells in children, at a time when the neural restraint placed upon the release of gonadotrophin releasing hormone lowers serum gonadotrophin and testosterone to undetectable levels. In this respect, AMH is more informative than inhibin, which is produced by both Sertoli and Leydig cells. The serum level of AMH declines soon after birth, at the end of the gonadotrophin surge [4]. AMH levels are not affected by human chorionic gonadotrophin (hCG) stimulation [2] and are decreased in hypopituitary children with gonadotrophin deficiency [5].

N. Josso
Unité de Recherches sur l'Endocrinologie
du Développement (INSERM)
1, rue Maurice-Arnoux
F–92120 Montrouge (France)

0301–0163/92/0388–0072
$ 2.75/0

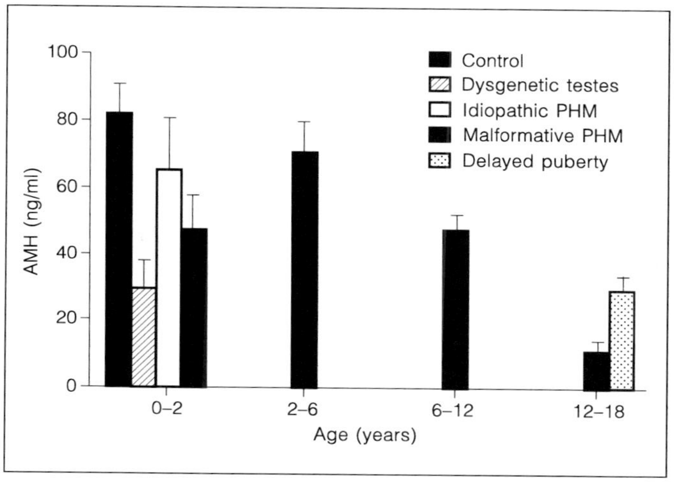

Fig. 1. Mean and variability (SEM) of serum AMH in 117 normal boys according to age: under 2 years (n = 33), 2–6 years (n = 30), 6–12 years (n = 41), and 12–18 years (n = 13). Also depicted are values found in children with various developmental disorders: testicular dysgenesis (n = 7), malformative male pseudohermaphroditism (n = 6), idiopathic male pseudohermaphroditism (n = 10) and boys with delayed puberty. From reference [2], with permission.

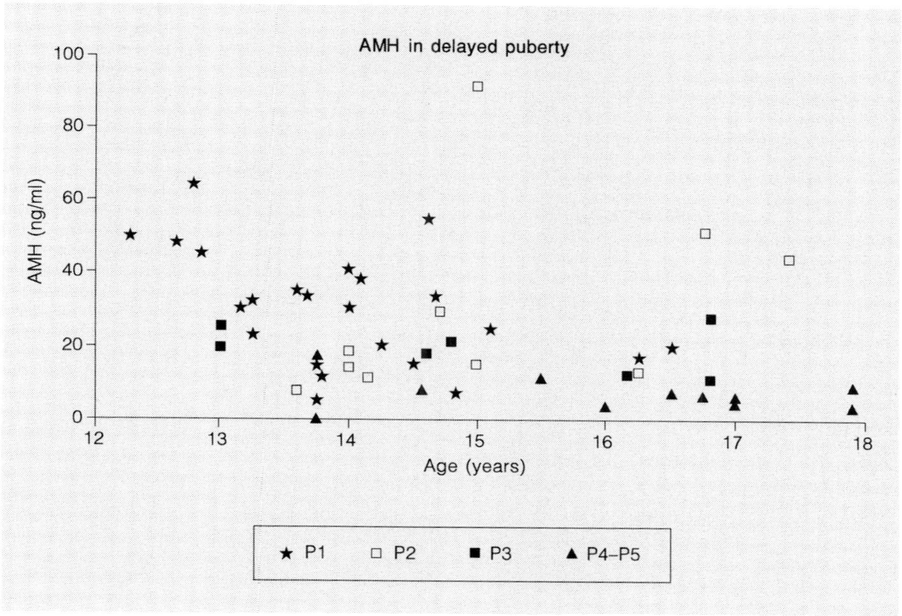

Fig. 2. Influence of pubertal maturation on AMH serum concentration in boys with delayed puberty. The pubertal stages correspond to Tanner's classification (P1 = no signs of pubertal maturation, P5 = full pubertal maturation). Pubertal maturation is associated with a decrease in AMH serum concentration. From reference [16], with permission.

AMH in Paediatric Endocrine Disorders

In clinical practice, it is not unusual to question the existence of testicular tissue in children. The problem arises in normally virilized children in whom testes cannot be palpated (fig. 3). Until now, assaying plasma testosterone was the only method of exploration. However, this method has the drawback that, after the newborn period, prolonged hCG stimulation is required to induce testosterone production by the testes. Assaying serum AMH requires no testicular stimulation (indeed no means of increasing AMH production by the testes is known at the present time). Also, as only the testes produce a measurable amount of AMH in children, no false-positive results due to adrenal hyperfunction or covert testosterone administration, for example, can arise. However, false-negative results are possible if severe testicular dysgenesis is present or the patient is affected with the persistent Müllerian duct syndrome. It should be stressed that AMH measurement is useful only in children well below the age of puberty, because in older children low AMH concentrations are not unusual.

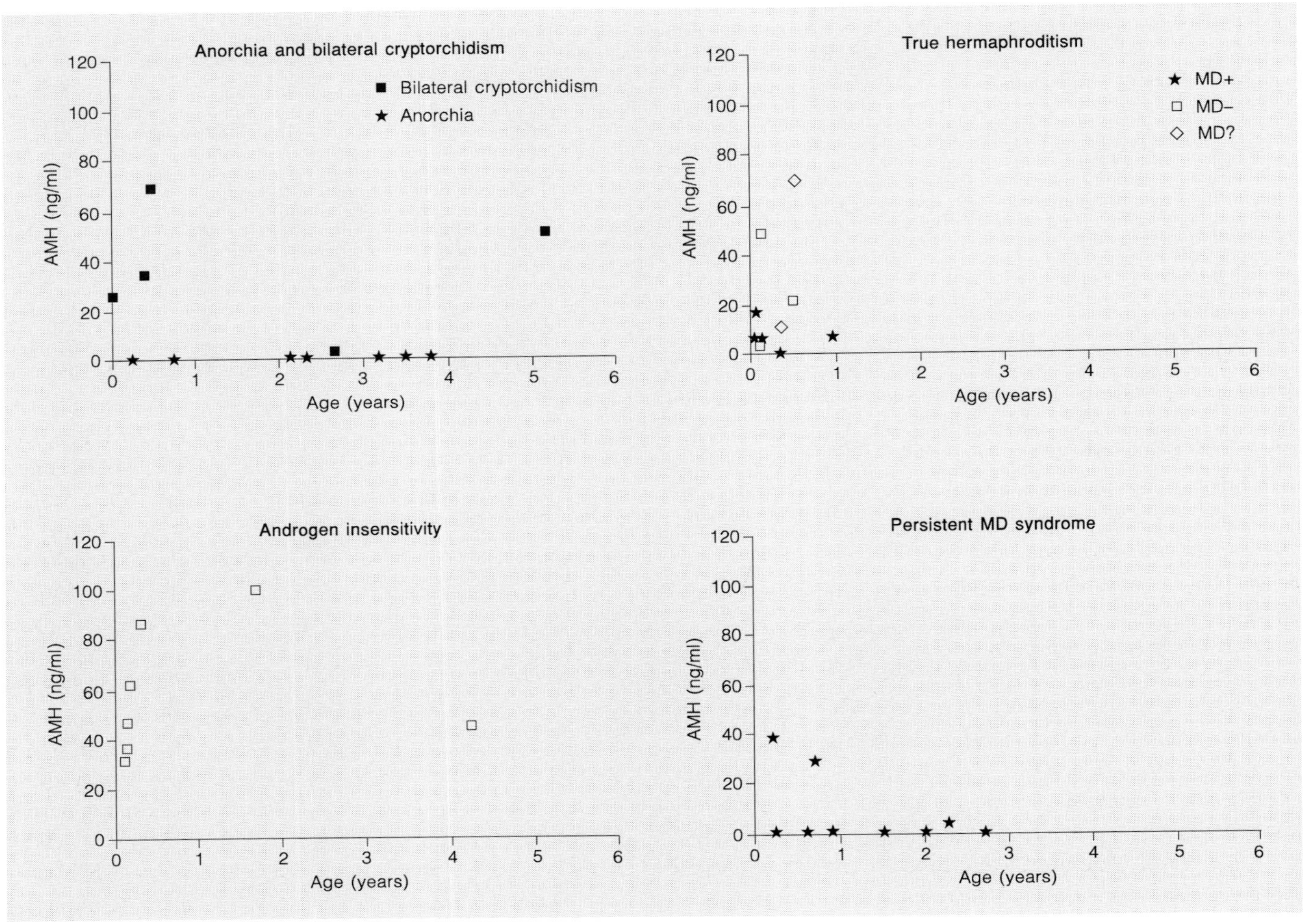

Fig. 3. Serum AMH values in sex ambiguity. Top left: AMH assay is usually able to distinguish between anorchia and bilateral cryptorchidism, except in a 2.5-year-old patient with severe gonadal dysgenesis. Top right: AMH serum concentration in true hermaphroditism. AMH concentration is usually decreased, only 2 of 10 patients had values within normal limits. MD+: A uterus and tube were present, at least unilaterally. MD–: Müllerian ducts were normally regressed. MD?: Müllerian status unknown. From reference [16], with permission.

AMH in Intersex States

AMH levels in various intersex states are shown in figure 3. In a recent study [2] we showed that serum AMH is significantly decreased in male pseudohermaphrodites with testicular dysgenesis compared with other forms of male pseudohermaphroditism. Long-term follow-up will show whether AMH values have a prognostic value, for instance in the prediction of fertility, in those patients raised as males. AMH values are normal in patients with androgen insensitivity. AMH measurement is also useful in sexually ambiguous XX infants, to discriminate between idiopathic female pseudohermaphroditism (where no testicular tissue is present) and true hermaphroditism. In true hermaphrodites, AMH levels are usually detectable, but low. In our series [6], of 10 hermaphrodites, only two had AMH serum values within normal limits. Anatomical evidence for Müllerian regression and serum AMH levels do not always correlate. Müllerian regression reflects testicular anti-Müllerian activity at the initiation of sex differentiation (at 8 weeks of fetal life), whereas serum AMH provides information on testicular function at the time of the study.

Persistent Müllerian Duct Syndrome

The persistent Müllerian duct syndrome (PMDS) is a rare form of inherited male pseudohermaphroditism, characterized by the presence of a uterus and Fallopian tubes in otherwise normally virilized males. Some years ago the diagnosis was usually made in adult or adolescent patients undergoing surgical repair of cryptorchidism or inguinal hernia. Because early treatment of undescended testes is now advocated, the incidence in children has increased in recent years.

PMDS is often associated with cryptorchidism, not because AMH has a direct effect on testicular descent, but because the testes are tightly linked to the Fallopian tubes. Generally in PMDS, the Müllerian derivatives are not fixed in the pelvis and are dragged into the inguinal canal by the descending testis. The inguinal hernia, called 'hernia uteri inguinalis' in the literature, contains the uterus and tubes. Clinically, there is a negative correlation between cryptorchidism and inguinal hernia on the same side. The testis and hernia are always palpable together, because of the tight attachment of the testis to the Fallopian tube. Gentle traction on the uterus draws the contralateral tube and testis into the inguinal canal. Traction is not always necessary; sometimes both testes are already in the same inguinal canal. This is known as 'transverse testicular ectopia' almost never encountered when cases of PMDS are excluded. More rarely, the uterus and tube are maintained in the pelvis by the round ligament, and the testes are in an 'ovarian' position. Clinically, the patients are bilaterally cryptorchid, and no inguinal hernia is present.

If there is no index case in the family, PMDS is not usually suspected prior to surgery for cryptorchidism or inguinal hernia. This creates practical difficulties, because the surgeon may be unacquainted with PMDS and unprepared to perform the difficult separation of vas deferens from the Müllerian derivatives. When, for any reason, PMDS is suspected prior to surgery, inguinal or pelvic sonography can be helpful.

Treatment should aim at preserving fertility. Testicular tissue differentiates normally in PMDS patients. If the testes are in a scrotal position, or if early correction of cryptorchidism has been carried out, the germ cell population is normal and is expected to undergo normal spermatogenesis. Fertility then depends on the preservation of the male excretory duct system. Sloan and Walsh [7] have stressed that total hysterectomy is dangerous because of possible injury to the vasa deferentia embedded in the uterine wall and to the epididymis, contained in the mesosalpynx. However, it is usually impossible to bring the testes into the scrotum if Müllerian derivatives are left intact, because the free segment of the spermatic cord is too short. This can be corrected by careful dissection of the cord, followed by salpingectomy and corporeal hysterectomy, leaving the fimbriae and cervix intact. In patients with transverse testicular ectopia, crossed orchidopexy gives good results.

AMH-Positive and AMH-Negative Forms of PMDS

PMDS is a heterogeneous disorder, involving either AMH or the Müllerian duct. Elucidating the etiology of PMDS is only feasible during childhood, when the testis normally expresses high amounts of AMH. A lack, or severe decrease, of testicular AMH production can be assessed by measuring the level of circulating AMH (fig. 3); it is probably due to an abnormality of the AMH gene.

When levels of circulating AMH are normal, a test of the anti-Müllerian activity of the testicular biopsy is required to distinguish between Müllerian duct insensitivity and an AMH gene mutation affecting the bioactivity but not the immunoreactivity of the molecule. This test gives valid results in children below the age of 2 years [8]. If the testicular biopsy is able to induce regression of the rat Müllerian duct, Müllerian duct insensitivity must be blamed for the occurrence of PMDS. Peripheral AMH resistance could be due to a receptor abnormality or to desynchronization between AMH production by Sertoli cells and the window of Müllerian duct sensitivity to AMH. In the human fetus, Müllerian ducts respond to AMH only before 8 weeks' gestation [9] and any delay in the initiation of AMH production by the fetal testis results in preservation of the Müllerian duct system. On the other hand, if the testicular biopsy does not induce rat Müllerian duct regression, a mutation leading to the production of an immunoreactive, but not bioactive, protein is the most likely cause.

Genetics of PMDS

PMDS is a genetic disorder, with 12 sets of siblings including one pair of identical twins [10] described in the literature. The anatomical position of the uterus, Fallopian tubes and testes is not genetically determined [11]. The mode of transmission of the disorder has been difficult to elucidate because, until recently, AMH-positive and AMH-negative cases could not be distinguished. Most family trees are compatible with the autosomal recessive, male restricted transmission expected in patients with a defect in the autosomal AMH gene [12], but an apparently sex-linked PMDS transmission has been reported in two families [7, 13]. The AMH status of these patients is unknown. X-linked transmission could be explained in the AMH-positive form if the gene for the AMH receptor, which may possibly be involved, was located on the X chromosome. Against this hypothesis is the fact that, in dogs, AMH-positive PMDS is transmitted as an autosomal recessive trait [14] and one would expect X-linkage to be conserved between species. The problem will be resolved when X-linked cases of PMDS become available for testing and the AMH receptor is cloned.

Several mutations of the AMH gene, associated with PMDS have been described in AMH-negative forms of PMDS. A nonsense mutation was described in a Moroccan family with three affected boys [11]. A guanine to thymidine transversion, at position 2096 in the fifth exon, changes a GAA triplet coding for Glu 358 into a TAA ochre termination codon interrupting translation and leading to a truncated AMH molecule, which can be visualized in culture medium of Chinese hamster ovary cells transfected with the mutated gene [11]. In another child, a patient of Drs Rosenthal and Loeff in Chicago, cytosine is replaced by thymine at nucleotide position 377, changing a CGG arginine codon to a TGG tryptophan codon. The substitution of tryptophan, a bulky aromatic residue, normally within the hydrophobic cores, is expected to constrain the secondary structure, thus affecting protein folding and stability. Finally, compound heterozygosity, associating a 14 bp deletion in one allele with a stop mutation in the other, was detected in a patient of Dr Maria New in New York [15].

Until now, allele-specific hybridization, performed with DNA from approximately 20 PMDS AMH-negative patients, has not revealed any mutational hotspots. This emphasizes the need for effective screening techniques to pin-point the defective DNA region. Understanding relationships between structure and function should help to elucidate the basic requirements for biological activity, particularly in the AMH-positive form of the disorder, which affects the bioactivity, but not the stability of the molecule.

References

1 Josso N, Picard JY: Anti-Müllerian hormone. Physiol Rev 1986;66:1038–1090.

2 Josso N, Legeai L, Forest MG, et al: An enzyme-linked immunoassay for anti-Müllerian hormone: A new tool for the evaluation of testicular function in infants and children. J Clin Endocrinol Metab 1990;70:23–27.

3 Josso N, Boussin L, Knebelmann B, et al: Anti-Müllerian hormone and intersex states. Trends Endocrinol Metab 2:227–233.

4 Burger HG, Yamada Y, Bangah ML, et al: Serum gonadotrophin, sex steroid, and immunoreactive inhibin levels in the first two years of life. J Clin Endocrinol Metab 1991;72: 682–686.

5 Swaenepoel C, Adamsbaum C, Brauner R, et al: Anti-Müllerian hormone serum levels are decreased in boys with congenital hypopituitarism. Pediatr Res 1991;35(Suppl S2):50–51 (Abstract).

6 Josso N, Vigier B, Magre S, et al: Anti-Müllerian hormone and gonadal development. Seminars Dev Biol 1991;2:285–291.

7 Sloan WR, Walsh PC: Familial persistent Müllerian duct syndrome. J Urol 1976;115: 459–461.

8 Donahoe PK, Ito Y, Morikawa Y, et al: Müllerian inhibiting substance in human testes after birth. J Pediatr Surg 1977;12:323–330.

9 Josso N, Picard JY, Tran D: The anti-Müllerian hormone. Rec Progr Hormone Res 1977; 33:117–160.

10 Weiss EB, Kiefer JH, Rowlatt UF, et al: Persistent Müllerian duct syndrome in male identical twins. Pediatrics 1978;61:797–800.

11 Guerrier D, Tran D, Van der Winden JM, et al: The persistent Müllerian duct syndrome: A molecular approach. J Clin Endocrinol Metab 1989;68:46–52.

12 Cohen-Haguenauer O, Picard JY, Mattei MG, et al: Mapping of the gene for anti-Müllerian hormone to the short arm of human chromosome 19. Cytogenet Cell Genet 1987;44:2–6.

13 Naguib KK, Teebi AS, Al-Awadi SA, et al: Familial uterine hernia syndrome: Report of an Arab family with four affected males. Am J Human Genet 1989;33:180–181.

14 Meyers-Wallen VN, Donahoe PK, Ueno S, et al: Müllerian inhibiting substance is present in testes of dogs with persistent Müllerian duct syndrome. Biol Reprod 1989;41:881–888.

15 Harbison MD, Magid MLS, Josso N, et al: Anti-Müllerian hormone in three intersex conditions. Ann Genet 1991;34:226–232.

16 Josso N, Cate RL, Picard JY, et al: Anti-Müllerian hormone: The Jost factor. Rec Progr Hormone Res 1992 (in press).

Horm Res 1992;38(suppl 2):77–81

I.A. Hughes
D.M. Williams
J.A. Batch
M.N. Patterson

Department of Paediatrics,
University of Cambridge, UK

Male Pseudohermaphroditism: Clinical Management, Diagnosis and Treatment

Key Words
Karyotype
Testes
Androgens
Hormone resistance
HCG stimulation

Abstract
Male pseudohermaphroditism (MPH) is a disorder of sexual differentiation whereby the external genitalia are at variance with a male karyotype and the presence of testes. Abnormalities of Leydig cell function are an important cause of MPH, but postnatal age must be considered when interpreting the testosterone response when HCG stimulation is used as a diagnostic test. Androgen insensitivity is also a common cause of MPH; the specific defect in androgen receptor function is currently the subject of intense study, using a combination of biochemical assays and molecular analysis of the androgen receptor gene. The treatment of MPH is influenced by genital tissue responsiveness to androgens and the technical complexity of reconstructive surgical procedures. There is a need for information on the outcome of MPH treatment regarding pubertal development, sexual performance and fertility.

Introduction

Male pseudohermaphroditism (MPH) refers to a disorder of sexual differentiation characterized by external genitalia which are incompletely masculinized in an individual with a 46XY karyotype, bilateral testes and male internal genital ducts. The term is used rather loosely to encompass a large number of possible causes, but MPH is clearly distinguishable from either female pseudohermaphroditism (virilized female external genitalia and a 46XX karyotype) or true hermaphroditism (the presence of testicular and ovarian tissue but a variable karyotype).

Causes of MPH

Normal androgen production and its transport and action at its target site is a fundamental prerequisite for adequate masculinization in the developing male. Reference to figure 1 indicates that a defect in any of the steps in this pathway may result in MPH. The possible causes are numerous [1] and the major groups are listed in table 1.

Decreased Androgen Production

In the male, congenital hypopituitarism is typically associated with micropenis but otherwise normally formed external genitalia. Hypoglycaemia resulting from adrenocorticotrophin (ACTH) deficiency is a common and urgent problem which has to be resolved.

Incomplete masculinization of the external genitalia is a manifestation of one of the steps in the pathway of androgen synthesis shown in figure 2. Most of the enzyme defects are common to both testicular and adrenal tissue; for example in 3β-hydroxysteroid dehydrogenase deficiency, the consequences of adrenal insufficiency are usually the dominant feature of the clinical manifestations. In contrast, 17β-

I.A. Hughes
Department of Paediatrics
University of Cambridge
Cambridge (UK)

0301–0163/92/0388–0077
$ 2.75/0

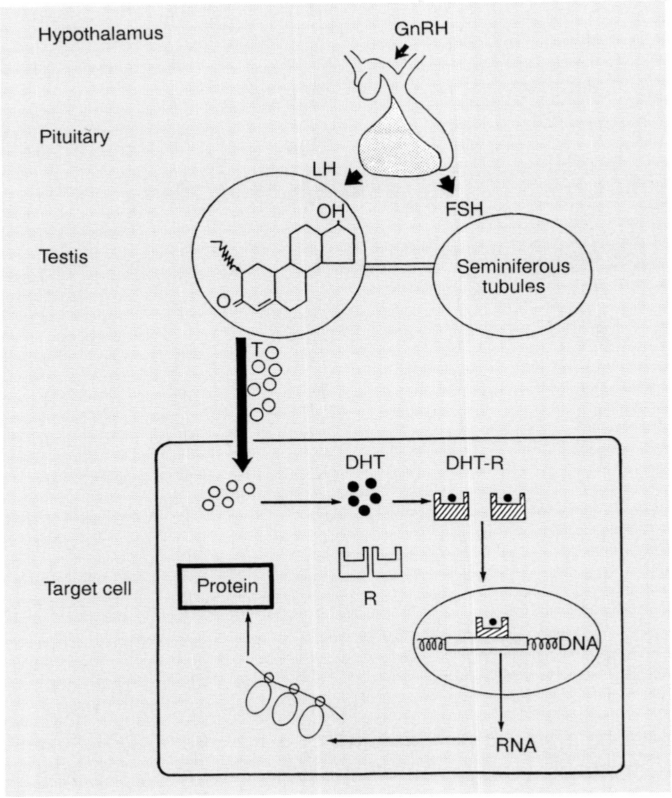

Fig. 1. Schematic pathway of androgen production and action. T = Testosterone; DHT = dihydrotestosterone; R = androgen receptor.

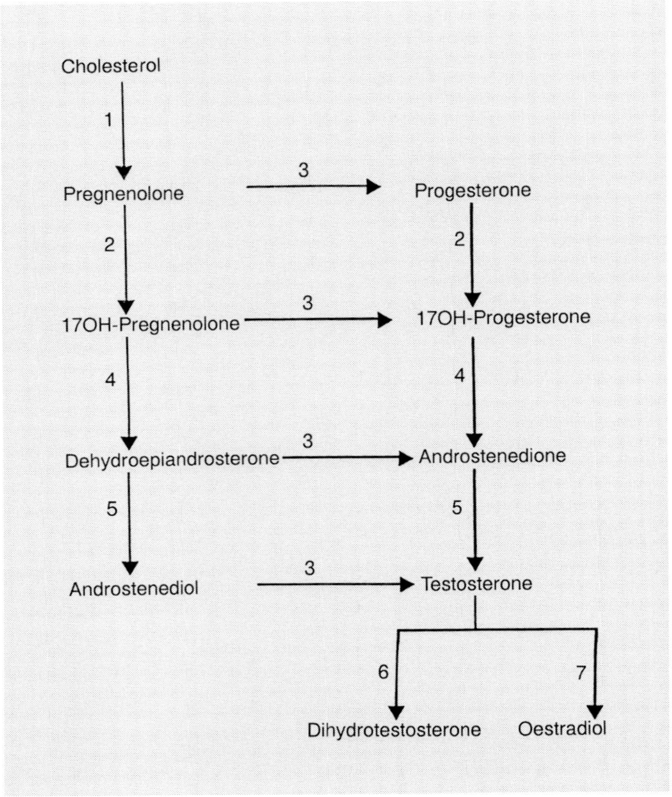

Fig. 2. Sex hormone biosynthesis in the testis. The numbers refer to the following enzymes: 20,22-desmolase (1); 17α-hydroxylase (2); 3β-hydroxysteroid dehydrogenase (3); 17,20-desmolase (4); 17β-hydroxysteroid dehydrogenase (5); 5α-reductase (6); aromatase (7).

hydroxysteroid dehydrogenase is a non-adrenal enzyme and is required for the conversion of androstenedione to testosterone. Males with a deficiency of this enzyme are severely undervirilized at birth and are usually reared as females. If the diagnosis is missed at birth, then quite profound masculinization of the external genitalia may take place at puberty. This is an intriguing event and does not explain why androgens do not have a similar biological effect in earlier fetal life.

Testicular dysgenesis is a vague term used to describe abnormal differentiation of the gonads during fetal life. This cause of MPH can only be confirmed by histological examination. The germ cells are poorly differentiated with immature tubules and no spermatogenesis. Leydig cells are often abundant, and the lack of adequate masculinization at birth is attributed to inadequate androgen production during the early critical period of fetal sex differentiation. There is a high risk of gonadoblastoma and germ cell tumours developing in dysgenetic testes [2].

Table 1. General classification of MPH

Decreased androgen production
Gonadotrophin deficiency
Leydig cell hypoplasia
Defects in steroidogenesis
Abnormal androgen metabolism
5α-reductase deficiency
Increased aromatase activity
Normal androgen production
Androgen insensitivity syndromes

Abnormal Androgen Metabolism

The principal circulating androgen, testosterone, acts as a prohormone since conversion to dihydrotestosterone (DHT) in certain target tissues produces an amplified androgenic effect [3]. The 5α-reductase enzyme responsible for the conversion is preferentially expressed in the fetal external genital anlagen during a critical period in male embryogenesis [4]. The clinical phenotype which presents at birth as a result of a deficiency in this enzyme, predictably has micropenis, perineal hypospadias, absent prostate and normal Wolffian structures [5]. What is also known, but not fully explained, is the profound virilization of the external genitalia in these individuals at the time of puberty.

It is theoretically possible that inadequate masculinization may arise because of enhanced conversion of androgens to oestrogens owing to the increased activity of the aromatase enzyme. Although the Sebright and Campine chickens represent animal models of such a phenomenon [6], the evidence that this may occur in man is not substantial [7].

Normal Androgen Production and Hormone Resistance

The final cause of MPH is hormone resistance. This is defined as either the lack of a biological response in a target tissue to normal or increased concentrations of the trophic hormone, or the requirement for an abnormally increased concentration of hormone to elicit the desired biological effect. Since Albright first alluded to the concept of end organ unresponsiveness in relation to parathyroid hormone action in pseudohypoparathyroidism [8], hormone resistance syndromes have been described for most of the major circulating hormones. The androgen insensitivity syndromes, associated with androgen resistance, contribute a major group of disorders leading to MPH. The complete form is characterized by normal female external genitalia. The partial forms of androgen insensitivity manifest phenotypically as a spectrum which ranges from mild virilization (e.g. isolated clitoromegaly) to a predominantly male phenotype with micropenis, abnormal scrotum and severe hypospadias. The eponymous descriptions applied to some male phenotypes are not useful and provide no information on causation. The term partial androgen insensitivity syndrome is often used rather loosely to describe a clinical phenotype which can also result from causes not associated with hormone resistance (table 2).

Hormone resistance is studied in vitro by ligand binding assays using specific target cells. In the case of androgens, cultured genital skin fibroblasts provide a useful system for analyzing androgen binding, both quantitatively and qualitatively [9]. The complete form of androgen insensitivity is usually binding negative, whereas in general the partial forms are binding positive. This distinction provides a useful starting point when devising a strategy for molecular analysis of the androgen receptor gene [10]. For example, receptor negative complete androgen insensitivity is typically associated with a mutation affecting those exons encoding the ligand binding domain of the androgen receptor protein. In contrast, the DNA binding domain encoded by two exons is more likely to be affected in the receptor positive form. The partial form of the syndrome is less clearly demarcated in the relationship between quantitative receptor binding and mutational analysis. It is likely that mutations in putative gene(s) other than the androgen receptor gene will be shown to explain some of the phenotypes in true partial androgen insensitivity.

Table 2. Disorders associated with micropenis and perineoscrotal hypospadias phenotype

3β-hydroxysteroid dehydrogenase deficiency
17,20-desmolase deficiency
17β-hydroxysteroid dehydrogenase deficiency
5α-reductase deficiency
Mixed gonadal dysgenesis
Dysgenetic MPH
True partial androgen insensitivity syndrome

Investigation

MPH often presents as ambiguous genitalia of the newborn. The most common cause of this problem (adrenal 21-hydroxylase deficiency) will have to be excluded, based on a normal plasma 17OH-progesterone level for age and a 46XY karyotype. There is no place for guesswork based on the appearance of the external genitalia. The usual signs are a micropenis with chordee, surrounded by a bifid scrotum, and a perineoscrotal hypospadias. The gonads may be palpable and are likely to be testes, though ovotestes are also a possibility. The nature of the internal genitalia can be determined by ultrasound examination, which should also be used to examine the renal tract for evidence of associated urological anomalies. There may be a utricle remnant, but the presence of Müllerian duct elements, such as a uterus, suggests dysgenesis of the testes as a possible cause of MPH.

An HCG stimulation test to assess Leydig cell function is a central component of the schedule of hormone investigations (table 3). Several factors will influence the results, including the postnatal age of the infant. Figure 3 depicts the pattern of plasma testosterone concentrations from birth to puberty, as adapted from data in the literature [11–13]. There is a striking surge in testosterone levels hours after birth, followed by a more gradual secondary increase in levels which peak at approximately 2 months of

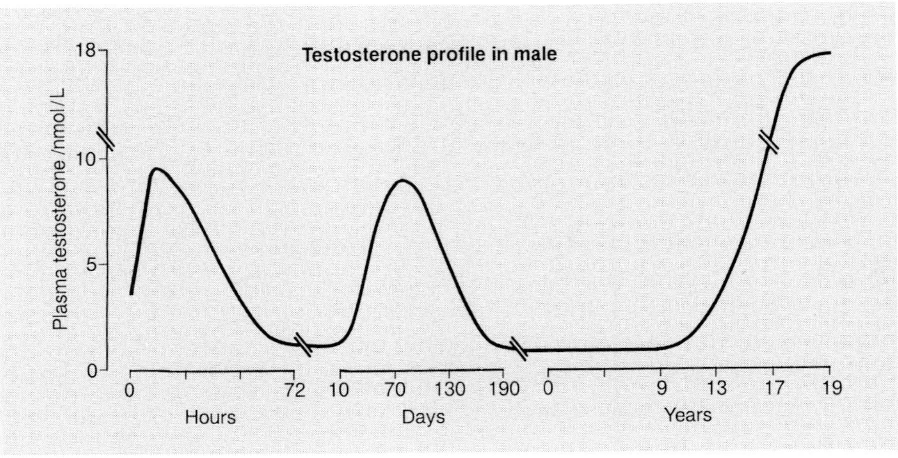

Fig. 3. Schematic profile of plasma testosterone levels in the male from birth to puberty (adapted from the literature [11–13]).

age. Testosterone concentrations fall to low prepubertal levels by 4–6 months of age and remain so until the onset of puberty. The basal and peak testosterone response to HCG stimulation will vary according to when the test is performed in relation to postnatal age. A standard protocol is three daily injections of 2000 units with a post-HCG sample collected 24 h after the last injection [14]. Occasionally it may be necessary to give the HCG injections over a longer period of time. An alternative protocol uses a single HCG dose of 5000 units.

It is not usually necessary to measure all the steroids listed in table 3. An adequate testosterone response virtually excludes a testosterone biosynthetic defect. In 17β-hydroxysteroid dehydrogenase deficiency, increased androstenedione in the face of decreased testosterone levels is the diagnostic marker. For 5α-reductase deficiency, the ratio of testosterone to dihydrotestosterone concentrations following HCG stimulation is a specific test for this enzyme defect [15]. Measurement of urinary steroid metabolites by specific chromatographic techniques is an essential adjunct, to define the precise enzyme deficiency in defects of testosterone biosynthesis and metabolism.

A normal testosterone and dihydrotestosterone response to HCG stimulation implies some defect in androgen action as a cause of MPH. When reconstructive surgery to the external genitalia is carried out, a genital skin biopsy for fibroblast culture can be obtained to study androgen binding in vitro. The results are used to determine which part of the androgen receptor gene is likely to contain a mutation. Blood samples for DNA extraction should be obtained from the index case and other relevant family members. In addition to the classic X-linked androgen insensitivity syndrome, isolated hypospadias can be familial and, if severe, this condition also warrants analysis of the androgen receptor. There is no evidence that simple, isolated hypospadias is associated in postnatal life with either a defect in androgen production or an abnormality in androgen action [16].

Table 3. List of steroids to measure in an HCG stimulation test

Plasma	17OH-progesterone
	17OH-pregnenolone
	Dehydroepiandrosterone (sulphate)
	Androstenedione
	Testosterone
	Dihydrotestosterone
Urine	Androsterone
	Aetiocholanolone
	Dehydroepiandrosterone
	16α OH-dehydroepiandrosterone
	Androstenetriol

Treatment

Management of the complete form of androgen insensitivity with normal female external genitalia is relatively straightforward. Gonadectomy is required at some stage. There is increasing preference for performing this procedure when the diagnosis has been established, rather than waiting until the signs of puberty are complete. Oestrogen replacement is required at the appropriate time.

MPH associated with abnormal genitalia presents a more difficult management problem. The decision on the sex of rearing is usually taken in close consultation with the surgeon. A trial of androgen treatment serves two purposes. Firstly, a response in terms of increased phallic growth indicates a certain degree of androgen responsiveness. Secondly, the reconstructive surgery carried out in hypospadias repair is technically easier to perform. Two or three monthly injections of testosterone (Sustanon, 25 mg) are usually sufficient. The precise details of surgical technique are not relevant, but the severe hypospadias with little foreskin tissue generally needs a mucosal graft and perhaps more than a one-stage procedure. In vitro studies of androgen binding and molecular analysis of the androgen-receptor gene have not provided sufficient information to predict reliably the longer-term response to androgens in those reared as males. The identification of a specific mutation is clearly of benefit in genetic counselling.

Patients with MPH caused by inadequate androgen production should respond adequately to androgen replacement. Parenteral treatment is commonly used, although oral preparations of androgen, such as mesterolone, are used in the longer term.

Conclusion

The outcome for patients with MPH should be assessed on the short-term success of corrective surgery to the external genitalia, adequate masculinization at puberty and thereafter, sexual performance and fertility in adult life. There is currently little information available on each of these three important components of the outcome of management in MPH.

References

1 Savage M: Clinical aspects of intersex; in Brook CGD (ed): Clinical Paediatric Endocrinology. 2nd edn. Oxford, Blackwell Scientific Publications, 1989, pp 38–54.
2 Savage MO, Lowe DG: Gonadal neoplasia and abnormal sexual differentiation. Clin Endocrinol 1990;32:519–533.
3 Grino PB, Griffin JE, Wilson JD: Testosterone at high concentrations interacts with the human androgen receptor similarly to dihydrotestosterone. Endocrinology 1990;126:1165–1172.
4 Siiteri PK, Wilson JD: Testosterone formation and metabolism during male sexual differentiation in the human embryo. J Clin Endocrinol Metab 1974;38:113–125.
5 Imperato-McGinley J, Guerrero L, Gautier T, et al Steroid 5α-reductase deficiency in man: An inherited form of male pseudohermaphroditism. Science 1974;186:1213–1215.
6 George FW, Wilson JD: Pathogenesis of the henny feathering trait in the Sebright bantam chicken. Increased conversion of androgen to estrogen in skin. J Clin Invest 1980;66:57–65.
7 Hemsell DL, Edman CD, Marks JF, et al: Massive extraglandular aromatization of plasma androstenedione resulting in feminization of a prepubertal boy. J Clin Invest 1977;60: 455–464.
8 Albright F, Burnett CH, Smith PH, et al: Pseudohypoparathyroidism – An example of 'Seabright-Bantam' syndrome. Endocrinology 1942;30:927–932.
9 Hughes IA, Evans BAJ: The fibroblast as a model for androgen resistant states. Clin Endocrinol 1988;28:565–579.
10 French FS, Lubahn DB, Brown TR, et al: Molecular basis of androgen insensitivity. Recent Prog Hormone Res 1990;46:1–42.
11 Corbier P, Dehennin L, Castarier M, et al: Sex differences in serum luteinizing hormone and testosterone in the human neonate during the first few hours after birth. J Clin Endocrinol Metab 1990;71:1344–1348.
12 Forest MG, Sizonenko PG, Cathiard AM, et al: Hypophysogonadal function in infants during the first year of life – I. Evidence for testicular activity in early infancy. J Clin Invest 1974; 53:819–828.
13 Winter JSD, Hughes IA, Reyes FI, et al: Pituitary-gonadal relations in infancy: 2. Patterns of serum gonadal steroid concentrations in man from birth to two years of age. J Clin Endocrinol Metab 1976:42:679–686.
14 Hughes IA: The gonads; in Handbook of Endocrine Investigations in Children. London, Butterworth, 1989, pp 110–129.
15 Imperato-McGinley J, Peterson RE, Gautier T: Decreased urinary C19 and C21 steroid 5-alpha-metabolites in parents of male pseudohermaphrodites with 5-alpha-reductase deficiency – detection of carriers. J Clin Endocrinol Metab 1985;60:553–558.
16 Evans BAJ, Williams DM, Hughes IA: Normal postnatal androgen production and action in isolated micropenis and isolated hypospadias. Arch Dis Childhood 1991;66:1033–1036.

Horm Res 1992;38(suppl 2):82–85

D. Aarskog

Department of Pediatrics,
University of Bergen, Norway

Syndromes and Genital Dysmorphology

Key Words
Aarskog syndrome
CHARGE association
Dysmorphology
Hypospadias
Opitz syndrome
Prader-Willi syndrome
Robinow syndrome
VATER association

Abstract
External and internal genitalia can be malformed by genetic and environmental factors without involvement of sex chromosomes or fetal gonads. Thus, genital dysmorphology may be part of many syndromes of various etiology, such as monogenetic disorders, autosomal chromosomal abnormalities and non-random malformation syndromes of unknown etiology. Genital dysmorphology may also occur as a result of teratogenic effects following maternal ingestion of synthetic progestins. The genital manifestations in all these syndromes occur more commonly in males than in females. Penetrance and expression of these abnormalities tend to show great variability.

Introduction

Most patients with intersex conditions are generally well formed, except for the genital abnormalities. The abnormal development of the genital organs in patients with intersex conditions can generally be explained by abnormalities in the constitution of the sex chromosomes, abnormal development of the gonads, and/or endocrine disorders. External and internal genitalia can also be malformed in the same way as other organs, such as the kidneys, heart and limbs, by genetic or environmental factors, without involvement of sex chromosomes or gonads.

General Principles of Dysmorphology

Establishing the diagnosis of a dysmorphology syndrome is an art of clinical recognition. This involves identifying, collecting, sorting out, and arranging a set of minor and some major anomalies into a recognizable pattern. Diagnosis by pattern identification requires familiarity with dysmorphology syndromes and requires experience and knowledge. The expression 'the more you see, the more you know' and 'the more you know, the more you see' accurately describes the process by which knowledge of pattern recognition develops. Physical and laboratory findings may also be included in the recognition process. For example, the finding of a micropenis and hypoglycaemia in a neonate with orofacial clefting should generate a prompt diagnosis of congenital hypopituitarism [1].

Most of the defects which make up a dysmorphic syndrome are minor anomalies with few or no functional or cosmetic consequences. The anomalies tend to occur in complex structures, such as the face, ears, hands and feet. In this context, the external genitalia of the male are more complex structures than those of the female. Accordingly, some kinds of genital abnormality occur more frequently in males than in females. Because of the close relationship of the genital and urinary organs, malformations of the sex organs are often combined with malformations of the urinary tract.

In general, the clinical diagnosis of a syndrome can not be made on the basis of a single defect, and, with rare exceptions, there is no obligate defect. It should also be borne in mind that variation in the expression of a given defect among individuals with the same syndrome is common.

D. Aarskog
Department of Pediatrics
University of Bergen
Bergen (Norway)

0301–0163/92/0388–0082
$ 2.75/0

Etiology

The known modes of etiology for dysmorphology syndromes include monogenic disorders (autosomal dominant, autosomal recessive and X-linked), chromosomal abnormalities and environmental teratogens. However, there still remains a large group for which the etiology has not been revealed. During the past two decades the number of recognized syndromes has greatly increased, and to help clinicians record them, electronic reference systems have been developed. One of these databases, POSSUM (Pictures of Standard Syndromes and Undiagnosed Malformations), now contains information on 1783 different syndromes. In 555 of these syndromes there are some defects involving the external genitalia; the majority of which involve the male organs. It should be noted that both under and over growth of the penis are regarded as dysmorphic features.

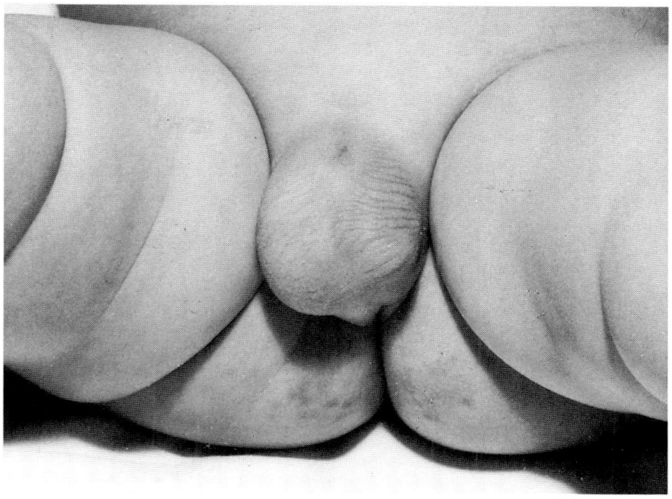

Fig. 1. Congenital absence of the penis in a 9-month-old boy.

Monogenic Disorders

Genital dysmorphology may be part of a number of genetic disorders. In general, both penetrance and expression of the genital manifestations in such syndromes show great variability. It is beyond the scope of this paper to give comprehensive coverage of all these conditions, and they will only be illustrated by a few examples. Extensive surveys of syndromes with relevant pictures and references are available in several recent atlases [2].

Robinow syndrome is characterized by short stature, short arms, hypoplastic genitalia and a characteristic face [3]. Some families have been reported with autosomal dominant inheritance and others with autosomal recessive inheritance. Since the face resembles that of a human fetus at 8 weeks, the descriptive term 'the fetal face syndrome' has been proposed. The genital hypoplasia consists of hypoplastic clitoris and labia minora in females, and micropenis in males. Absent penis has also been observed. Isolated absence of the penis is a rare condition (fig. 1).

Opitz syndrome, or the hypertelorism-hypospadias syndrome is an autosomal dominant syndrome [4]. Affected females have normal genitalia, whereas males have various degrees of hypospadias. In more severe cases there are also anomalies of the scrotum with clefting and anterior displacement of the penis.

Aarskog syndrome is an X-linked disorder characterized by short stature, hypertelorism, short nose with anteverted nostrils, long philtrum, and genital dysplasia [5]. The distinguishing feature of the syndrome is a scrotal fold extending dorsally and surrounding the base of the penis. This characteristic genital manifestation has been referred to as shawl or saddle scrotum (fig. 2). Cryptorchidism and inguinal hernia are also major features.

Autosomal chromosomal disorders can be associated with malformations of the genital tracts and external genitalia. Hypospadias, split scrotum, cryptorchidism, uterus duplex bicornis or unicornis, and vagina septa may occur in the classical autosomal chromosome disorders. Ambiguity of the genitalia which raises doubts as to the sex of the patient has been described [6].

Hypoplasia of the male external genitalia is one of the main features of the Prader-Willi syndrome. It has been shown that approximately 50% of patients with Prader-Willi syndrome have a deletion of the proximal part of the long arm of chromosome 15, or the 15q11-q13 region. Recently, studies using molecular markers have demonstrated that the deleted chromosome is derived from the father. In patients with Prader-Willi syndrome who have no visible chromosome deletion, marker studies have disclosed two copies of the mother's chromosome 15 [7]. Thus, it seems to be lack of the 15q11-q13 part of chromosome 15 coming from the father which produces Prader-Willi syndrome.

Environmental or teratogenic factors might cause abnormal development of the genital organs. Two years before the thalidomide tragedy, in 1958, Lawson Wilkins and his colleagues reported a series of 14 newborn girls who had been virilized by maternal use of synthetic progestins in the early weeks of pregnancy [8]. The masculinization of

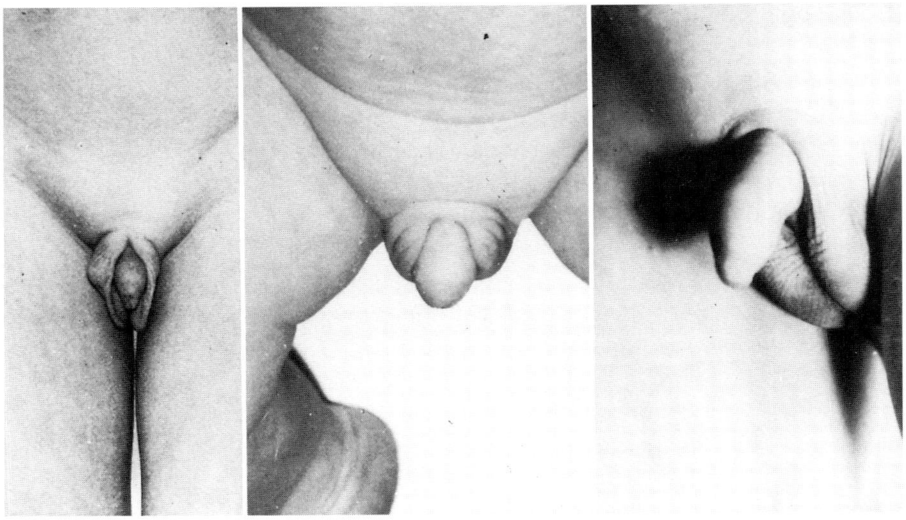

Fig. 2. Variations in the genital manifestation of Aarskog syndrome. Note clefted scrotum and scrotal fold extending round the base of the penis.

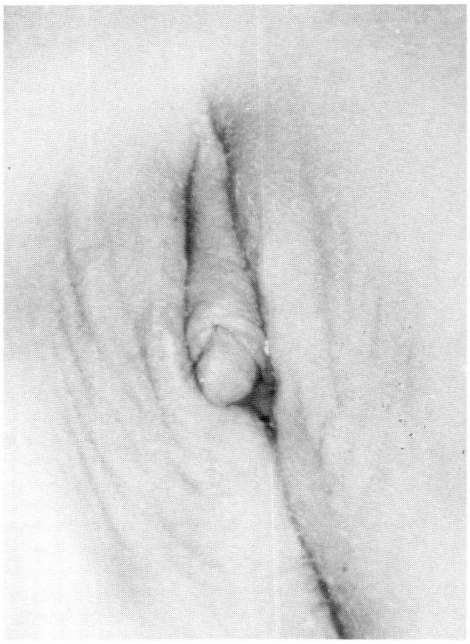

Fig. 3. Clitoral hypertrophy in a 6-year-old girl whose mother had been treated with synthetic progestin during early pregnancy.

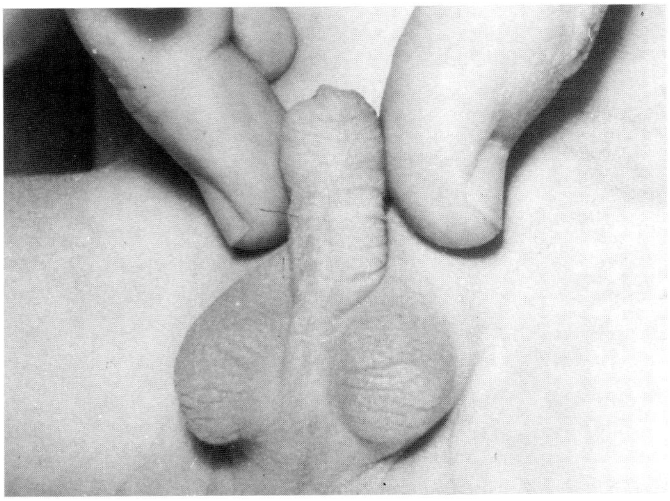

Fig. 4. VATER syndrome in a newborn boy. Note bifid scrotum with caudal displacement and distal thickening of the penis.

the external genitalia involved enlargement of the clitoris and various degrees of labial fusion. In most cases, the clitoral hypertrophy regressed spontaneously within the first year of life, but in some cases the enlargement persisted into childhood (fig.3).

In the late 1960s several reports suggested an association between maternal progestin treatment and the development of hypospadias in the male fetus. In a personal study of 11 cases of hypospadias with a history of maternal progestin ingestion, there was a relationship between the position of the urethral meatus and the week of gestation when progestin treatment was started. The more proximal openings occurred in the children of mothers treated in the first month of pregnancy [9].

The explanation of this seemingly paradoxical effect of progestin on the female and male fetuses may be explained by the fact that progestins and dihydrotestosterone compete to bind at the same receptor. In the female, this results in a slight androgenic signal resulting in virilization. In the male, progestin reduces dihydrotestosterone binding and thus prevents full masculinization.

The non-random malformation association syndromes are designated by acronyms, to aid in remembering their cardinal features. The VATER association originally included Vertebral defect, Anal atresia, Tracheo-Esophageal fistula and Radial limb defect. Later the association was expanded to include cardiac defects, renal defects and genital defects [10]. The most characteristic genital defects are clefting of the scrotum and anterior displacement of the penis (fig. 4).

The CHARGE association consists of four or more of the following defects: Coloboma of iris and/or retina, Heart defect, Atresia choanae, Retarded growth, Genital hypoplasia and Ear anomalies. In males, genital hypoplasia with micropenis is a distinct feature [11].

References

1 Knudtzon J, Aarskog D: Growth hormone deficiency associated with the ectodactyly-ectodermal dysplasia-clefting syndrome and isolated absent septum pellucidum. Pediatrics 1987;79:410–412.

2 Jones KL: Smith's Recognizable Pattern of Human Malformation. Philadelphia, WB Saunders 1988, 4th edn.

3 Butler MG, Wadlington MB: Robinow syndrome: Report of two patients and review of the literature. Clin Genet 1987;31:77–85.

4 daSilva EO: The hyperterlorism-hypospadias syndrome. Clin Genet 1983;23:30–34.

5 Aarskog D: A familial syndrome of short stature associated with facial dysplasia and genital anomalies. J Pediatr 1970;77:856–861.

6 Fluge G, Myking A, Aarskog D: Male pseudohermaphroditism in a patient with E-trisomy syndrome. Acta Paediatr Scand 1973;62: 440–444.

7 Nicholls RD, Knoll JHM, Butler MG, et al: Genetic imprinting suggested by maternal heterodisomy in non-deletion Prader-Willi syndrome. Nature 1989;349:281–285.

8 Wilkins L, Jones HW Jr, Holman GH, et al: Masculinization of the female fetus associated with administration of oral and intramuscular progestins during gestation: Non-adrenal female pseudohermaphroditism. J Clin Endocrinol Metab 1958;18:559–585.

9 Aarskog D: Maternal progestins as a possible cause of hypospadias. N Engl J Med 1979;300: 75–78.

10 Apold J, Dahl E, Aarskog D: The VATER association: Malformations of the male external genitalia. Acta Paediatr Scand 1976;65: 150–152.

11 Davenport SLH, Hefner MA, Mitchell JA: The spectrum of clinical features in CHARGE syndrome. Clin Genet 1986;29:298–310.

Author Index

Aarskog, D. 82
Batch, J.A. 77
Boulware, D. 47
Calender, A. 16
Caprio, S. 47
Clemmons, D.R. 37
Gertner, J.M. 41
Gooren, L.J.G. 51
Hawkins, J.R. 62
Haymond, M.W. 44
Hofman, M.A. 51
Holl, K. 24
Horber, F.F. 44
Hughes, I.A. 77
Josso, N. 72
Lenoir, G.M. 16
LeRoith, D. 1
Padberg, B.C. 24
Patterson, M.N. 77
Raue, F. 31
Riley, W.J. 9
Roberts, C.T., Jr. 1
Saenger, P. 36
Scherbaum, W.A. 7
Schröder, S. 24
Schuffenecker, I. 16
Shemer, J. 1
Sizonenko, P.C. 50
Swaab, D.F. 51
Tamborlane, V. 47
Underwood, L.E. 37
Voutilainen, R. 66
Williams, D.M. 77
Zink, A. 31

Subject Index

Aarskog syndrome 82
Addison's disease 9
Adrenal phaeochromocytoma 24
Anabolism 37
Androgens 77
Anorchia 72
Anti-Müllerian hormone 66
Autoantibodies 9
Autoimmune diseases 9
CHARGE association 82
Dysmorphology 82
Endocrine 1
Evolution 1
Fat distribution 41
Gender 51
Gene 16
Genetics 16
Gonadotrophins 66
Growth hormone 41
HCG stimulation 77
HLA-DR antigens 9
Hormone resistance 77
Human growth hormone 44
Hypospadias 82
Hypothalamus 51
Inhibins 66
Insulin secretion 47
– sensitivity 47
Insulin-dependent diabetes mellitus 47
Intersex states 72
Karyotype 77
L-[1-^{14}C]leucine 44
Leucine 44
Medullary thyroid carcinoma 24, 31
MEN 1 31
MEN 2a 31
MEN 2b 31
Metabolism 41
Mucocutaneous candidiasis 9
Mucosal ganglioneuromatosis 24
Müllerian inhibiting factor 72
– – substance 72
Multiple endocrine neoplasia 16, 24
Muscle mass 37
Neurocrine 1
Nitrogen balance 37
Opitz syndrome 82
Ovary 66
Pancreatic islet cell tumour 31
Parathyroid hyperplasia 24
– tumour 31
Peptide hormones 1
Persistent Müllerian duct syndrome 72
Phaeochromocytoma 31
Pituitary tumour 31
Prader-Willi syndrome 82
Predictive screening 16
Prednisone 44
Protein synthesis 44
Proteolysis, *L*-[1-^{13}C]leucine 44
Puberty 47
Review 9
Robinow syndrome 82
Screening 31
Sertoli cells 72
Sexual orientation 51
Sipple's syndrome 31
Somatomedin-C 37
SRY 62
Steroidogenesis 66
TDF 62
Testes 77
Testis 66
– determination 62
VATER association 82
Wermer's syndrome 31
XX males 62
XY females 62

World Review of Nutrition and Dietetics (ISSN 0084–2230),
Vol. 70
Series Editor: A.P. Simopoulos, Washington, D.C.

Metabolic Control of Eating, Energy Expenditure and the Bioenergetics of Obesity

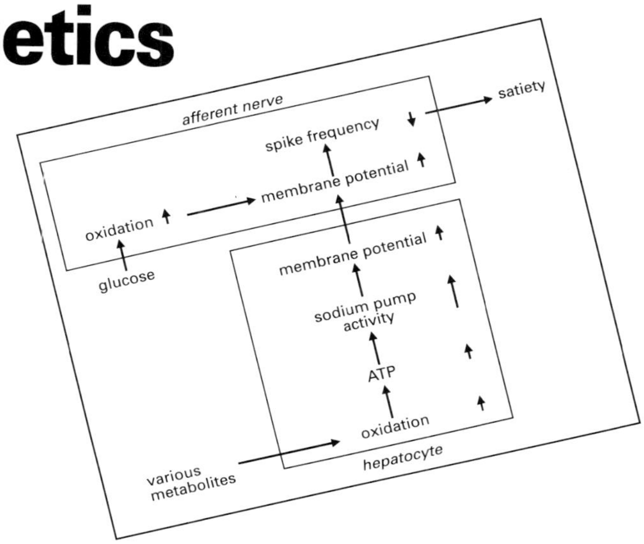

Editor:
Artemis P. Simopoulos

This volume brings together the most up-to-date reviews on three subjects of major importance to the study of obesity. It opens with a comprehensive description of the metabolic control of eating. The paper includes sections on eating and energy balance, meal-taking behavior, effects of circulating fuels on eating, and the various controls that exist such as control of eating by hepatic metabolism, pancreatic hormones, metabolic sensors in the brain, as well as metabolic cues and taste perception. The second paper authoritatively reviews the theory and practice of calculating energy expenditure and fuel selection based on indirect calorimetry and tracer methods. The final paper on the bioenergetics of obesity is a major review of research from 1981–1991.

A valuable single source of information, this book will interest physiologists, biochemists, nutritionists, dietitians, physicians interested in obesity and clinical nutrition, as well as researchers in the fields of pharmacology, exercise physiology, membrane biochemistry, endocrinology, metabolism and genetics.

Contents

Simopoulos, A.P.: Preface
Langhans, W.; Scharrer, E.: Metabolic Control of Eating
Elia, M.; Livesey, G.: Energy Expenditure and Fuel Selection in Biological Systems: The Theory and Practice of Calculations Based on Indirect Calorimetry and Tracer Methods
Olowookere, J.O.: The Bioenergetics of Obesity Syndrome

Fields of Interest

Nutrition; Metabolism;
Biology for Physicians, Dietetics, Endocrinology

World Review of Nutrition and Dietetics, Vol. 70
Metabolic Control of Eating,
Energy Expenditure and the Bioenergetics of Obesity
Editor: Simopoulos, A.P. (Washington, D.C.)
XII + 176 p., 33 fig., 27 tab., hard cover, 1992
SFr. 235.– / DM 281.– / £ 102.20 / US$ 188.00
Prices subject to change
US $ price for USA, £ price for UK, DM price for FRG only
ISBN 3-8055-5595-4

Frontiers of Gastrointestinal Research
(ISSN 0302–0665), **Vol. 21**
Series Editors: P. Rozen, Tel Aviv; C. Scarpignato, Parma

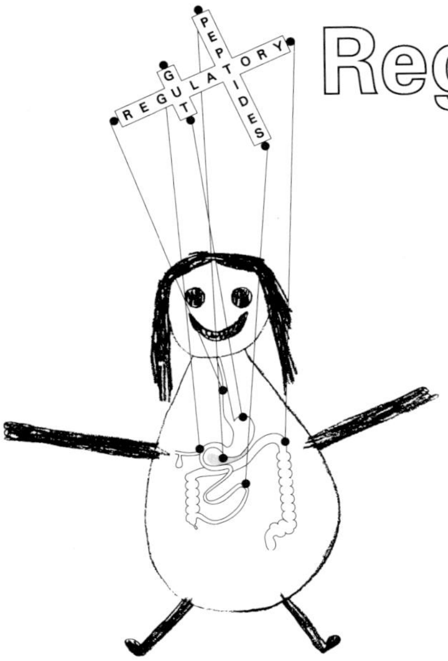

Regulatory Gut Peptides in Paediatric Gastroenterology and Nutrition

Editors: P. Heinz-Erian, J. Deutsch, G. Granditsch

Growth and function of the gastrointestinal tract are highly dependent on specific interactions of regulatory gut peptides (RGP) with their target tissues. This timely volume compiles state-of-the-art reviews on the existence, the cellular mechanisms of action and the biological functions of these peptides as well as their significance in health and disease during the paediatric period. The opening section of the book provides an overview of the distribution, biochemistry and physiology of RGP. The second section relates specific functions of the normal gastrointestinal tract, such as transit, digestion, absorption and secretion, to the action of RGP and summarizes what is actually known about these functions in normal children. The impact of RGP on growth and nutrition in the normal child as well as the influence of feeding on their release is dealt with in the third section. The final section extensively discusses the significance of RGP for paediatric gastrointestinal diseases and gives an outlook on the now rapidly emerging therapeutic potential of this class of compounds.

Addressing all aspects of RGP in children and indicating gaps in current knowledge, this book is essential reading for paediatric gastroenterologists, neonatologists, paediatricians, endocrinologists, oncologists and physiologists.

Contents

Distribution, Biochemistry and Physiology of Regulatory Gut Peptides in the Gastrointestial Tract
Bishop, A.E.; Polak, J.M.: The Neuroendocrine System of the Gut: Visualization · *Laburthe, M., et al.:* Gut Peptide Receptors and Signal Transduction in Intestinal Epithelium: State of the Art · *Christophe, J., et al.:* Gut Peptide Receptors and Signal Transmission in the Exocrine Pancreas and in the Pancreatic Acinar Cell Line AR 4-2J · *Said, S.I.:* Biological and Physiological Actions of Regulatory Gut Peptides in the Gastrointestinal Tract · *Brown, J.C.:* Metabolic Effects of Regulatory Peptides of the Gastrointestinal Tract

Effects of Regulatory Gut Peptides on Basic Functions of the Normal Gastrointestinal Tract
Milla, P.J.: Regulatory Gut Peptides and Gastrointestinal Transit · *Fölsch, U.R., et al.:* Digestive Function and Regulatory Gut Peptides with Special Reference to the Role of Cholecystokinin · *Krejs, G.J.:* Intestinal Absorption and Secretion: Role of Regulatory Gut Peptides in Man · *Heinz-Erian, P.:* Gastrointestinal Function in Healthy Children: Significance of Regulatory Gut Peptides

Regulatory Gut Peptides: Role in Paediatric Growth and Nutrition
Lebenthal, E.; Lu R.B.: Ontogeny of Regulatory Gut Peptides · *Milner, R.D.G.:* Regulatory Gut Peptides and Growth · *Aynsley-Green, A., et al.:* Regulatory Gut Peptides in the Perinatal Transition Period · *Koldovský, O., et al.:* Possible Role of Milk-Borne Peptide Growth Factors for the Breast-Fed Infant

Regulatory Gut Peptides in Paediatric Gastrointestinal Disease
Nelson-Piercy, C., et al.: Gastrointestinal Endocrine Tumours during Childhood · *Milla, P.J.:* Regulatory Gut Peptides in Hirschsprung's Disease and Other Gut Motility Disorders · *Hyman, P.E.; Eysselein, V.E.:* Regulatory Peptides in Inflammation, Ulceration, and Tissue Repair: Inflammatory Bowel Disease and Peptic Ulcer Disease · *Aynsley-Green, A., et al.:* Gut Regulatory Peptide Profiles in Acute Gastroenteritis and Necrotising Enterocolitis in Infancy · *Buchanan, K.D.; Johnston, C.F.:* Regulatory Peptides in Coeliac Disease and Other Mucosal Intestinal Disorders · *Teufel, M., et al.:* Regulatory Gut Peptides and Cystic Fibrosis · *Hill, I.D.; Lebenthal, E.:* Therapeutic Significance of Regulatory Gut Peptides in Childhood

Fields of Interest
Gastroenterology; Pediatrics; Endocrinology; Biochemistry, Hepatology, Nutrition, Oncology, Perinatal Medicine, Physiology, Popular Medicine

Frontiers of Gastrointestinal Research, Vol. 21
Regulatory Gut Peptides in Paediatric Gastroenterology and Nutrition
6th Annual Meeting of the GPGE, Goldegg/Salzburg, May 1991
Editors: Heinz-Erian, P. (Munich); Deutsch, J. (Graz); Granditsch, G. (Vienna)
VIII + 264 p., 41 fig., 15 tab., hard cover, 1992
SFr. 248.– / DM 297.– / £ 107.90 / US$ 198.50
US$ price for USA, £ price for UK only (subject to change)
ISBN 3–8055–5549–0

Pediatric and Adolescent Endocrinology (ISSN 0304–4254), **Vol. 21**
Series Editor: Z. Laron, Petah Tikva/Tel Aviv

Editors: C. Levy-Marchal, P. Czernichow

Epidemiology and Etiology of Insulin-Dependent Diabetes in the Young

Explores important facets of the diabetic puzzle

Concomitantly with the great advances made in genetic markers in diabetes, it has been observed that the incidence of diabetes in general, and of childhood diabetes in particular, seems to be on the increase but differs markedly among various populations. This timely volume brings up-to-date our knowledge of the factors that interact in the etiology of insulin-dependent diabetes mellitus (IDDM) from an epidemiological perspective. An exhaustive collection of data from the network of IDDM incidence studies around the world is presented and the role of the HLA system in the genesis of IDDM is emphasized. In addition, the question of IDDM screening in families and normal populations is approached not only from a methodological and statistical point of view but also from an ethical perspective.

As the first publication devoted to the epidemiology of insulin-dependent diabetes in the young, this book is essential and stimulating reading for pediatricians, diabetologists and epidemiologists.

Contents

Methodological Aspects: Follow-Up and Case-Control Studies
Follow-Up and Case-Control Studies: Study Design and Statistical Aspects · The Swedish Childhood Diabetes Study: Methodological Aspects

Incidence Studies

Descriptive Epidemiology
The North-South Gradient of the IDDM Incidence in Europe: Fact or Fiction? · Incidence of IDDM Outside Europe · The Incidence of Childhood IDDM in Various Ethnic Groups in Israel: A Population-Based Study – 1989 · Incidence of IDDM in Children in Finland and Estonia · The Case of Sardinia

Ethnic Groups and Migrant Studies
Epidemics, Migrants and the Death of the Pancreas · Epidemiology of Diabetes in Polynesia and New Zealand. Child Health Research Unit · Incidence Rate of Childhood IDDM in Latvia 1983–1989 · Comments from the Chairman

Clinical and Biological Studies
Clinical and Laboratory Features in Diabetic Children at the Time of Diagnosis: Results from the French Incidence Study · Comments from the Chairman

Genetics
Lessons on the Etiology of Insulin-Dependent Diabetes from Twin Studies · New Tools for HLA Studies · Use of HLA Information in IDDM through the MASC Method · HLA Population Genetics · Comments by the Chairman

Prediction - Epidemiological Aspects
Prediction of Insulin-Dependent Diabetes in Siblings of Newly Diagnosed Diabetic Children: The Finnish Experience · Prediction of Insulin-Dependent Diabetes. 1. Family Studies – 2. The General Population · Prevalence of Islet Cells Antibodies in French Children from Background Population · Discussion · Comments by the Chairman

Etiology
Nutritional Triggers of IDDM · Is Viral Infection an Initiating Factor for IDDM? · Effects of Breast-Feeding and Cow's Milk Consumption on Incidence of Type 1 Diabetes Mellitus · Comments by the Chairman

Fields of Interest

Biochemistry, Endocrinology; Pediatrics; Diabetes, Epidemiology, Genetics, Immunology, Nutrition, Preventive Medicine, Public Health, Statistics

Pediatric and Adolescent Endocrinology, Vol. 21
Epidemiology and Etiology of Insulin-Dependent Diabetes in the Young
Symposium on Epidemiology and Etiology of IDDM in the Young, Paris, May 1991
Editors: Levy-Marchal, C.; Czernichow, P. (Paris)
XII + 242 p., 44 fig., 38 tab., hard cover, 1992
SFr. 240.– / DM 287.– / £ 104.40 / US$ 192.00
US$ price for USA, £ price for UK only (subject to change)
ISBN 3–8055–5521–0

KARGER